Objects in Mirror
Are Closer Than They Appear

◆

Objects in Mirror Are Closer Than They Appear

◆

Inside Brain Injury

Sol Mogerman

People with Disabilities Press,
Stanley D. Klein, Ph.D., Series Editor
iUniverse, Inc.
New York Lincoln Shanghai

Objects in Mirror Are Closer Than They Appear
Inside Brain Injury

All Rights Reserved © 2001, 2006 by Sol Mogerman

People with Disabilities Press,
Stanley D. Klein, Ph.D., Series Editor
iUniverse, Inc.
an imprint of iUniverse, Inc.

iUniverse books may be ordered through booksellers or by contacting:

iUniverse
2021 Pine Lake Road, Suite 100
Lincoln, NE 68512
www.iuniverse.com
1-800-Authors (1-800-288-4677)

Credit for Graphic: Sol Mogerman

ISBN-13: 978-0-595-20942-2
ISBN-10: 0-595-20942-4

Printed in the United States of America

For
Gundula, Aaron, Reidar, Om, and Ian

Contents

Acknowledgements

I would like to acknowledge the many people who have helped me through my recovery and supported the writing of this book. Among them have been: Dr. Barry Jones (for saying the right thing at the right time), Dr. Mariko Tanaka (for seeing me through my transformation as a counselor), My Clients (for instructing me) Frieda Mogerman (for doing what mothers do best), Trudy Beaton (for believing in this book), The Denman Island Writers Group (for constructive criticism), Diane Davis (for editing the manuscript), Michael Flynn (for computer help), Sally Peterson at iUniverse (for helping me through the publishing process), Karen Graham (for helping format the manuscript), Michael E. Phelps, UCLA School of Medicine (for use of PET scan), Brian Grogan (for photography), Keith, Bentley, Mike, Bryce and John (for putting up with my whining and helping me keep sane), and mostly, the untiring love, support, and encouragement of my wife and children.

Introduction to First Edition

One of the main reasons we are able to imagine how others feel is because of our ability to compare and substitute like experiences for those we have not had ourselves. We use this ability when we empathize with our fellow human beings. I thought I could empathize with anyone using my powers of extrapolation until I was faced with trying to understand what it feels like to have suffered a brain injury. The interesting point of this exercise in attempted empathy was that the person with whom it was most difficult to empathize with—was myself.

The only experience I can think of that comes close to resembling the separation from self that occurs with brain injury, is the relief that I have felt upon waking up from the reality of a disturbing dream into the familiarity and comfort of my bedroom in "real" life. This feeling is usually accompanied by the thought "Boy, am I glad I'm Here!" With brain injury you yearn to wake up from its disturbing reality to the familiarity and comfort of your "real" life, but find that you can't, no matter how hard you try.

This book tells two stories. It gives my personal account of brain injury and puts forth the lessons I learned from my own recovery and those of my clients. My story is in the first part of the book ("Objects In Mirror Are Closer Than They Appear") and the lessons are in the second ("Inside Brain Injury"). You may chose to read both or either one alone; in any order or whichever you feel best suits your needs. It is my hope that this book provides you with the opportunity to experience what it is like to sustain a brain injury and gives you the understanding of how you can participate more effectively in your own recovery.

Introduction To Second Edition

It has been twenty years since my brain injury, seven since writing of the story of my recovery, and four since its publication as "Objects In Mirror Are Closer Than They Appear". I have come to believe that there is no end to the process of recovery from brain injury and have experienced a remarkable and unexpected return of ability and sense of self since the first publication of this book. The return of my seemingly lost ability to play the guitar happened to me in such an unexpected yet logical manner that I feel compelled to share the story of its restoration with my readership in this edition. Therefore the Epilogue of the first edition is replaced by Chapters 33–41 in keeping with the revelation that recovery is an infinitely progressive process that only appears finite when one stops to look at it in retrospect.

Prologue

"me—having the idea that I knew myself—that was me!"

–Stephanie, 17-year-old survivor of brain injury

How can we know who we are when we are not able to create and project meaningful ideas about ourselves that we receive back as reflections of our place in the world? We *can't*—and anyone who has suffered a brain injury has known the truth of it.

This story is about losing one's image in the mirror of the mind. It begins with the catastrophic trauma of serious physical injury unexpectedly transforming a friendly and nurturing world into one of utter desolation and betrayal. The power of such an experience can create a psychotic break. This break is positively regulated by the body as it rushes to catch up with the violent change of condition. Assuming consciousness is maintained, and disassociation not too great, one still can know *where* and *who* one is. A brain injury, however, fundamentally alters the very mirror of reality, which we are virtually dependent upon to know ourselves. Once this mirror is compromised in any degree, physical and psychological forces immediately arise to begin the painstakingly subtle process of repair and restoration.

This process is never ending. The journey begins at 12:30 AM on November 28, 1985.

Part I

Objects In Mirror Are Closer Than They Appear

CHAPTER 1

WAKE UP CALL

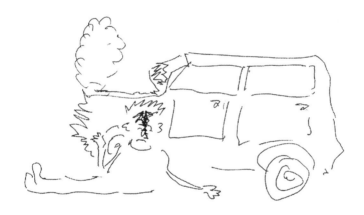

Dancing the edge, how easy to skirt the tyrant of convention. How fresh the creation of space and how light the load of joy.

This guy is a plodder—I play guitar so much better than he does. I'll bet he thinks he's cool. This really isn't much fun. I'm probably incurring huge karmic debt feeling this way. Did I invite him over only to show off my musical prowess?

Pride hung over the foothills as truncated clouds brushing the road with treachery.

They love me. They pay me to play music. I've finally arrived. It took moving to Canada to find my audience. God! This is sweet. I can't wait to get home. It must be cold out there—the road feels icy. I'm glad we got those studded tires.

Whoa! What's that guy doing on my side of the road? Just keeps on coming—No where to pull off without rolling the car and I'd have to walk home and get it towed out—too much trouble. I'll just let him get back over on his side—but the lights just keep on coming. I'd better pull over as far as I can without falling off the shoulder.

Here comes the crunch. This car's like paper. Man, what a blow. Stunning my head and legs. Hurts—Oh Oh…The engine's smoking. I'll be burnt to a crisp. I saw cars burn to nothing when I was a fireman. This baby might blow—and I'll never get to see my little boy grow up. Got to get out!! At least the window still rolls down—but the door's jammed. "Hey man, could you open the door?" Didn't even try! What's he laughing at? Ha Ha—Ho Ho. Guess I'll have to get out myself—don't want to burn up in here—out the window easy does it—Yow!! that's sharp!! I'll have to stay on the ground and drag myself away from that smoking car. There's something really wrong with my legs. Can't stand up. And it hurts to breathe. Too much pain!

God! I wish an ambulance would come. Is he trying to start his truck?

"Hey, brother. Don't leave me! That's inhumane. Call an ambulance!"

I'm really in trouble here! These guys smell like booze. They're acting like they don't even see me—like I'm not even here.

God this feels awful—I bet they wish I'd die.

"Hey! Call an ambulance!!"

The ground's cold and there's sticky blood in my eyes—Boom! Boom! What's that pounding background music?—like in a horror movie. Where's the ambulance? I'm okay! I'm okay!

But this is really a big deal. I've had a life changing car wreck and I'm really hurt! My life is on a pivot. Boom! Boom!

Got to keep awake! This is not a dream! I'm afraid if I wake up I'll die!

Taking forever. Where is that ambulance? I could really die of cold out here—Boom! Boom!

Why are those guys still laughing? Ha Ha—Ho Ho. I'd like to drop them in a pit and walk by to leave them there to suffer down in the darkness.

Okay, Thanks—someone's pressing on my forehead. Where are my glasses? Off-duty fireman. Where'd you come from? Thanks man—you say they're coming? You called them? Came from down the road? Who called you? That blanket feels good. Where are my glasses? I'm okay, just smashed up—can't stand—sorry for the blood. Hey, what's your name?

Bright lights. Strong arms. Yeah, I'm okay. Legs hurt—can't stand—I wish I was in my truck. Big 4X4 ex-army rig.

What do you drive? Oh yeah? Pretty cool. You guys got to call my wife as soon as possible. Tell her I'm okay—meet me at the hospital.

Okay, do your best. I'll just wait till the X-rays—and I'm okay—just my legs and chest hurt. Thanks for sewing up my head. When do you think I can get out of here?

Hey Babe. I'm okay. Just messed up a bit—I'll be out soon. Don't worry.

What's that guy hollering about? I recognize that laugh! That's one of the drunks! Guess he got a bit hurt too! Poor bastard hurt his shoulder. Who does he think he is carrying on like that?

God! What now! They want me to keep blowing into this plastic tube till the balls float! X-rays showed I bruised my lung and they want to keep it strong or I can't get out of here or something. What a drag! Also showed two cracked ribs and a broken ankle so I'll have to get an operation to get the ankle pinned. They won't do anything for the ribs. They hurt like hell! Guess I'll miss tomorrow's show and maybe some more after that!

So I got this cast on and now I have to leave the Intensive Care Unit. I like it here—I get lots of attention—sort of makes up for the road.

Now I'm really stuck in here with some old guys who are reading Reader's Digest. Not a very classy scene—really stupid. I want to get out of here so bad. Even I.C.U. was better than this.

I gotta piss but they won't let me walk on my cast yet, so I have to use this plastic pan with these old guys in here. God, this is bad—can't do it here.

Screw'em! I'll use those crutches and make it to the toilet—may be better standing up.

Whoa. Gotta sit down. Right Now.

Thanks for the chair. *Where did you come from?* Nurse slid that chair under me just in time—she must have been watching.

God—everyone looks so concerned! Had a stroke? That's okay, I'll get over it—I heard the guitar player from "Littlefeat" had one and he's playing again. It's just part of the trip.

But my left arm doesn't work! Like its sewn on and stuffed with crumpled up newspaper. *It's not mine!*

This may be serious—now they want to put me back in I.C.U.—looks like I got my wish!

I feel like a baby—everyone's freaked out about me having another stroke. Now they want to send me to a bigger hospital for an angiogram.

I feel so fragile—*who am I?*

Wait and wait. I'm thirsty but for some reason they won't give me water—only ice cubes. Hmm—dead horses hanging from the ceiling—how gruesome.

Wow! Check out that light show! What kind of test is this?

Okay, so my carotid artery looks like an accordion bellows—They figure it was struck in the wreck and created a clot to stop the blood flow to my brain.

What? Spend the night here with these dead horses? And the guy next to me with a brain tumor? What kind of hell have I landed in here? They're going to cut the poor guy's head open tonight. Luckily they're not going to cut me open, but want to send me back home to see a neurologist. I wonder what he can do for me?

Hey, this guy looks like Bozo the Clown with his funny hair sticking out on the sides. He is bald on top and has a fuzzy beard! Even though he's going to tell me the straight poop about my condition, I will always think of him as *Bozo*.

"There's not much I can do for you right now—you have already begun to heal your brain through your natural healing powers."

Yes! That is exactly what I want to hear!—a validation that I really am okay and will get better! Hey! Bring that guy back!

Everything is so hard to do—I am crying and feel like a baby. It is impossible to think about getting up and being a person again. I don't seem to know where the world stops and I begin.

CHAPTER 2

R2D2 VS. THE GALACTIC EMPIRE

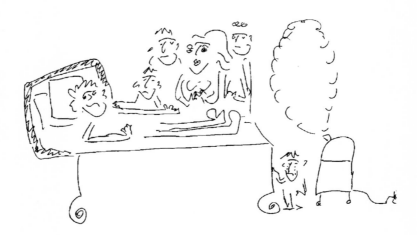

I feel like I'm floating. Even my wife and kids are strangers. The only real thing in my world seems to be the upbeat heart throb of the Bob Marley tape pumping into my ears through the headphones of the fancy new Walkman my wife bought me—*with what money?*

I yearn to be submerged in a cold stream and washed of my confusion. Instead I am plagued by stupid dry hospital air. When I ask for open windows a nurse tells me proudly that the hospital is sealed shut, and the climate is controlled by a computer in the basement.

I scream about how dry it is and they give me a little humidifier that looks like R2D2 from "Star Wars". It seems to help a bit and I make them keep it on 24 hours a day. At night, I imagine my little robot doing battle with the Galactic Empire so that I can breathe.

It is hard to relate to people. I don't feel at all like myself. The first bowel movement I take feels like I am passing a large steamship that is anchored to the very core of my body.

Now they want me to roam the ward in a wheelchair in order to get my strength back. I am so lopsided paralyzed that when I push with my arms I go in weak circles in the hallways. I get lost as soon as I leave my room. Somebody is always behind me cajoling "that's good!"…"keep pushing!"—*where did they come from?*

I finally find the TV room and don't like the color of the vinyl furniture. It doesn't matter. I can't sit down on it anyway. The TV is playing a show about an old woman who is riding in a train. I lickity split become her and can't follow the plot—even though I have somehow managed to absorb the reality of the show from a frightening perspective.

I find the whole experience very unsettling and want to go out into the hall to find my room somewhere.

The trip back takes me past the only window low enough for me to see out of in the whole ward. This is the first time I have been able to glimpse the outdoor world. There is snow all over the cars in the parking lot and, for the first time since my entry, I am glad to be in a warm building.

In the lot I see a big 4X4 Land Cruiser and decide that when I get my insurance settlement I want one so that the next time a drunk driver hits me head on, I will be protected by a car with some solid size. Somehow I know that lack of money, which usually plagues me, will not be an issue. It feels natural to be dependent and I forget what worrying about survival is like.

My wife has brought in my electric guitar (without amplifier) for me to try to play. I suppose she thinks it will help me get better faster because guitar playing is so much a part of my life. It is like holding a 2X4. I don't know what to do with it.

What is this? I was born knowing how to play the guitar. Now I seem to know less than I did before I was born! I thought it was like riding a bicycle—once you know how you never forget. *I have forgotten the unforgettable.*

My main desire is to get out of this place. I guess they are keeping me here in case I have another stroke. I wonder what good it will do to be here longer? If I have another stroke, I will just be more messed up or maybe die. I could do that anywhere.

CHAPTER 3

OVER MY DEAD BODY

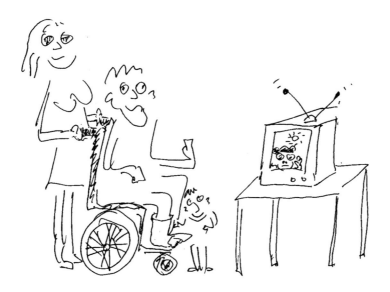

Finally they are letting me go home! My wife has rented a big four door Pontiac to drive me home. I am afraid it won't make it up the mountain in the snow—much less up the driveway.

It does. I never let her drive before.

Three young men have come up from California to visit my sons. They will carry me up the stairs into the house on a portable commode the hospital has loaned us—Pretty undignified way to enter Rome!

I can't seem to relax. Being at home is not much better than being in the hospital—I haven't snapped back to myself yet—and my ribs still really hurt. Life is pretty strange and painful.

My mother has come up from California to help the family. She is overly attentive and treats me like a baby. I don't care. Usually I would be all over her for hovering—Now I just don't care. I have settled in my little boy's room—*who is sleeping with my wife?*

Someone has given us an old black and white TV to help me convalesce. I fought off owning one for the last 25 years. "Over my dead body!" I used to say. Well they got pretty close.

Now I can scoot down the stairs, on my butt, to the basement where I keep my tools and sit by the wood stove that I welded together myself—from plates of 1/4-inch steel that I found along side the road. I was resourceful and skilled in the old days. My wife blindfolds me and brings me various things to identify with my left hand. A sparkplug, socket wrench, hammer, wire brush? Shit this is hard. I start to cry in frustration and throw the brush across the room. My wife comes back laden with more mysterious objects for me to identify. Sometimes I have a small victory. Yes that's a screwdriver. Big deal! The screwdriver was easy.

I like to hobble over to the workbench and look at my chainsaws. Sometimes I pick them up and heft them. The big firewood saw is heavy. I might drop it—but could I pull the rope and make it start? Luckily I put up twelve cords this summer before I got wrecked. I often sit by the wood stove in the basement and daydream about having my powers back.

Hanging around in the house is driving me crazy. The big picture window in the front room looks out on the valley below. What are those unicorns doing in the front yard? They are floating above the snow and lights are shooting from their hooves.

CHAPTER 4

WOULD YOU BUY A CAR FROM THIS MAN?

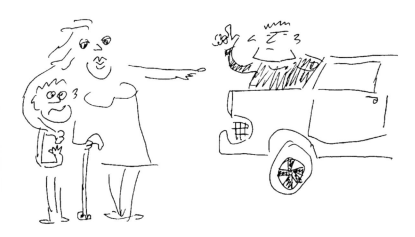

The rental car is going back and we need another rig. My mother is loaning us some money to buy a new car—something big with four-wheel drive. My wife is the test driver in the lots we go to because I am still unable to drive. It makes me mad! I'm the one who's bought all our cars so far. I feel like a wimp sitting next to her as she tries out the cars and the car salesman jokes about me being a gimp—but what the hell? I can't drive—so I let her do it, and his jokes don't sink in—I have no self-image. For the first time in my life I can afford to buy a decent car—and I can't drive it.

So we are buying a beautiful silver Jeep Cherokee Chief. I take home all the pamphlets, after the fact, pore over them at the table, and begin to develop rapprochement with my role as a man of property.

Now to drive my new car! The seat doesn't quite feel like it fits my body. I am profoundly uncomfortable. Again, like with the guitar, I am shocked that something that has been so comfortable and a part of me for the last 25 years feel so weird and foreign. At least the mechanics of driving haven't left me! I am still able to manipulate the clutch, gas, brakes and steering enough to make the car go, turn, and stop.

But the seat still doesn't feel quite right no matter how I fiddle with the adjustments. Neither does my ability to make judgments concerning traffic flow patterns.

When I am confronted with situations that require creative decisions about the rules of the road, like stopped school buses with flashing lights, road crews, and unmarked intersections, I choke up and make rash and impulsive choices about when to proceed. I am ignoring flashing lights (on school buses) and hand held road signs, which are there to direct me, because they break my flow and are *in my way*. Stoplights are also impediments and I have to tell myself over and over—"green, green, green", or "red, red, red" before driving through or stopping.

My family hates to drive with me and we have lots of fights in the car with them yelling at me while I try to defend the rapidly eroding illusion of my expertise as a driver.

CHAPTER 5

ROCK BOTTOM

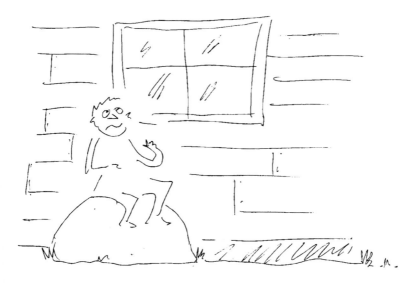

I have driven enough and we have scraped together enough money to take a trip back to California in the new car to visit our old community and my mother.

I seem to drive better as soon as I cross the Canadian border and hit the interstate highway. This is probably because there are fewer new decisions facing me in the chess game flow of highway driving.

I am always trying to feel like my old self and drive with the window down and my bare arm resting on the open window frame—just like in the old days.

I still don't feel right, not quite in sync with the car—and *never* comfortable in the damn seat.

Something is happening in my face and my left hand feels disconnected again. My lip is fluttering. It doesn't seem to affect my driving. I tell my wife what I am experiencing and she reassures me that maybe the feeling is coming back to the areas of my body affected by the stroke. I want to believe her and anxiously wait for the twitching to pass—which it does.

We are pleased to find that the people who bought our property in California are on vacation and we can stay in our old house, which we built and lived in for thirteen years before we came to Canada. This trip is the first time we have come back to the home we so recently left. It is emotionally overwhelming to be in the house I built with my own hands. I go to bed crying with an indescribable sweetness in my heart. I have a sense of complete surrender and sleep like a baby.

I am deeply grieved having left behind so much of myself, which it seems I will never be able to recover. I want to crawl into the womb of my old life and be born like I was. Most of my friends treat me like I used to be and I feel like a fraud.

Visiting a friend in town I am interrupted by a policeman who has followed me at the request of a gas station attendant I have forgotten to pay. It is obvious that my non-payment was an innocent oversight and I am embarrassed when my friend explains that the reason for my forgetfulness was due to the fact I had recently suffered a brain injury. He didn't have to say that!

We drive down to my mother's in Berkeley.

I thought that visiting the house I was raised in might help me discover my old self.

There is a rock in the yard I used to sit on as a child and, with a stick jammed in a crevice, pretend that I was driving a steamroller by moving the stick back and forth. I am drawn to this rock because it keeps bubbling up in my mind like a vision coupled with a good feeling. I seek this rock out with the vain hope that when I sit on it everything will be like it was. It is not so. No magic happens in or around my old family home. I am sad and go through the motions of visiting with my mother with little joy.

CHAPTER 6

SHAKE RATTLE AND ROLL

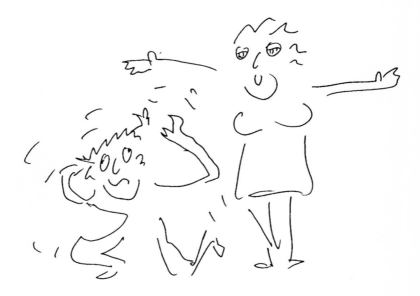

The drive back to Canada is uneventful except for the intense summer heat and I arrive home much as I was before.

Back home I am out in the woods checking one of our shallow wells for water level with a tape measure. As I am prying the heavy concrete lid back in place with a large crowbar I feel muscles flutter in my face, neck and left shoulder. This is not terribly remarkable and I wait for the fluttering to stop. It continues out of control and runs down into my left arm, which seems to be twisting up towards my back, and feels like it is being torn from my body by an invisible giant.

My wife looks questioningly at me but I cannot speak to reassure her that I am okay. Not because my mouth is affected in any way but because the words won't come to my lips. It is like they are stuck way back in my brain. I am terrified and fall to the ground, which catches me gently in its soft earthy arms.

My wife thinks I have suffered a heart attack and runs to the house to call our four sons out to the woods to say good-bye to their father. I feel like I am not going to die but still can't speak to tell every body that I am okay.

My sweet boys cradle me in their arms and kiss me and say they love me. One or two of them are crying. Someone finally has the presence of mind to run to the house and call an ambulance, which drives up into the woods to load and cart me off to the hospital.

They check me over for a heart attack and decide it must have been something else. It has been almost exactly one year since my stroke.

The doctors get smart and figure out it must have been a seizure. I don't really realize the ramifications of this diagnosis and, as usual, let them do their trip on me. This means anti-seizure drugs (Dilantin), which they deem to be the least complicated because I only have to take it once a day.

Dilantin proves to be a nightmare for me and I wander down the hallway of our house not knowing my right from my left side. I also break out in a bright purple rash all over my body, which burns tremendously.

My wife helps me into the bathtub where I soak in lukewarm water waiting to get some relief from the rash. I look down at my body and it looks wasted and purple. I have never looked so emaciated—and in color too!

We finally give up when the rash persists and decide to go back to the hospital. Because neither my physician, who in my opinion is worthless, or *Bozo*, whom I respect, are available, I am stuck with an emergency doctor who smells like stale pipe tobacco and makes the brilliant deduction that I am allergic to Dilantin. He also correctly assesses that I am completely freaked out and prescribes a sub-lingual *(I like that word)* tranquilizer, which gives me relief from the fear and confusion that I am feeling. I never thought modern medicine had so much to offer.

I am also put on a new anti-seizure medication (Tegretol) because the possibility of more seizures is a real threat. This new medication will take a few weeks to work itself into my system before it will be effective. I am supposed to see *Bozo* when he comes to town and get my dose adjusted for maximum protection.

Bozo figures my weight and prescribes 900 mgs of Tegretol starting me out on 300 and building me up slowly so that my body can adjust without debilitating side effects. He also tells me that the seizure might have been a one-time event and, until we know more about my condition, I must stop driving and using power tools—also stay off the roof and *don't swim alone.*

I am devastated—what is there left for me to do? I will be completely cut off from my old life. No music. No driving. No work. No play.

I am in a state of denial about the prospect of the seizures returning. The Tegretol seems to be holding them off or they won't be coming back anyway—or I am in between attacks. The side effects from 300 mgs don't seem to be more than minor drowsiness and cold sores in my mouth.

I am continuing to drive my car and use my big chainsaw. It feels great to "get back to normal". My wife is always after me to stay off the roof. Maybe she knows something I don't!

Things seem to be going great. I am involved in a big firewood-gathering project with a neighbor. It is fun to push my old 4X4 to the limit and build my strength back. I have even picked up a bit of work clearing the woods at a local hot springs in exchange for tub time, which I really enjoy.

One evening, after a day of cutting firewood, the neighbor and I are unloading my truck into his woodshed when the hand of hell once again grabs me by the shoulder. This time I swoon into my friend's arms. He gently lowers me to the ground where I quickly recover.

At first I am not too upset about this second seizure but after some time realize that it heralds real restrictions on the activities that I equate with getting better. I am overwhelmed by depression and make another appointment to see *Bozo* the neurologist.

Bozo looks me square in the eye and tells me that I have epilepsy as a result of the scarring of my brain from the stroke and that it will *not*, no matter how I wish it, go away. He also indicates that it is time to boost the Tegretol. I accept the treatment order and swear off driving for the prescribed year because I realize how dangerous it would be to be over-taken by a seizure while on the road.

The boost to 900 mgs is not as easy as I hoped. The side-effects seem to push my depression way out of control. No matter how I try, I am flattened by a mood, which saps all the joy from my life. I am also dazed, confused, and antagonistic towards any well-meaning attempts from others to help me.

I tell *Bozo* my complaints and he does not believe that the Tegretol could be affecting my mood so. I beg him to try to regulate my dosage so that it isn't so debilitating. He tries to reassure me that my body will eventually become accustomed to the drug and I will not be bothered by the side effects anymore. He also suggests that I try to decrease my intake to the point where the seizures are held off. Unfortunately there is no cut and dried scientific method for establishing this point. I must reduce it myself until the symptoms go away. This means that I may experience more seizures during the process. I hate the idea of having more seizures and am in a constant state of anxiety about it.

Then *Bozo* hits me with another of his show stopping quotes: "In a few years, you will look back upon all this as a bad dream!" Yes! That is exactly what I want to hear. I will be healed! I am healing! Thank You *Bozo*! Thank You God! Thank You Body!

In spite of the good news I am still dreadfully depressed and spend most of my time sitting at the table with my head in my hands. My wife is fed up and is trying to get me to do something with my life. We are on Welfare—money is very hard to come by and the insurance company is trying to starve us out for a smaller settlement. Our lawyer is a prince, but even he can't push the process any faster. He also tells me that the insurance company has spies watching me to make sure that I can't do what we are saying I can't do in the lawsuit. I find myself almost slowing down my recovery to accommodate the lawsuit. I know this is deeply wrong, but it seems the inevitable result of the adversarial system, which is supposed to compensate me for the wrongs perpetrated against me.

CHAPTER 7

FALSE START

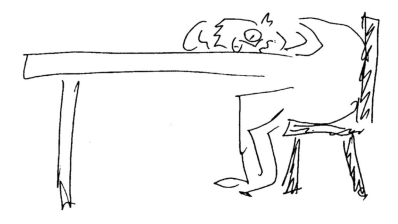

The kids keep going to school and are making a life for themselves ski-ing and watching TV. Nothing turns my crank but, for some reason, I am forcing myself to read.

One book, "Memories, Dreams and Reflections" by Carl Jung, is hold-ing my attention. It is actually doing much more than just holding my attention. It is exactly right for me now in my life and is infusing me with the excitement of *being* Jung himself. I feel I am actually living Jung's life and participating in his process as an innovative and groundbreaking psychologist. I want to do the very same thing with my life. It is the first time since my accident that I have been excited about anything!

Okay! So What? I am excited about a book. How can I do anything about it if I spend my days sitting at the table with my head in my hands?

My wife senses this change and pushes me to make an appointment at the local community college to see a career counselor. It takes a long time to get in because the counselor is very busy. This bums me out and I feel a million miles away from making anything happen. It all seems too slow and cumbersome to handle.

The counselor is a burnt out old guy who either doesn't have the savvy or energy to help me kindle the spark of excitement, which has begun to change my life. He prescribes a book called "What Color Is Your Parachute" and sends me home with the recommendation to buy it, follow its instructions, and come back to see him in a month. What he doesn't realize is that the prospect of buying a thirteen-dollar book pushes me farther back into depression because I don't think I am worth it. But I buy it anyway. I have no choice.

The book has a series of pages I am supposed to fill in like a work-book. This greatly turns me off because I have hated workbooks ever since elementary school. Still, I manage to scribble in enough pages to make the book tell me I want to be a psychologist like Jung. The book is useless. What I really want is someone to cheer me on!

Next time the counselor is smart enough to realize that I think I know what I want to do with my life. He now shows me some educational choices I have including a distance education program which could get me a Bachelor's of Social Work from the University of Victoria. This is not the psychology or counseling program I hope for but it will have to do. I sign up and wait for the books to come.

The first course is mildly interesting and the books are boring. I diligently write the papers and apply myself to forming the attitude of a social worker. The papers are hard to write and I struggle with our old typewriter. Lo and behold, someone somewhere thinks my papers are worth A's and I head off into the next course thinking that I might really become a social worker.

Course number two looks a bit better and demands more creative input asking me to write an in-depth paper on the subject of my choice. I choose Native Land Claims in B.C. because, as an American, I am fascinated with the fact that the relationship between natives and the white man is not a book closed by genocide like it is where I come from in California. I get bogged down in research and fearfully see the deadline for the paper's completion closing in on me. Figuring that distance education does not provide me with the encouragement I feel I need to get over the stall in my paper, I drop the course and fall deeper into depression.

Now I have no direction—it can only get worse.

CHAPTER *8*

SAME WAY EVERY DAY

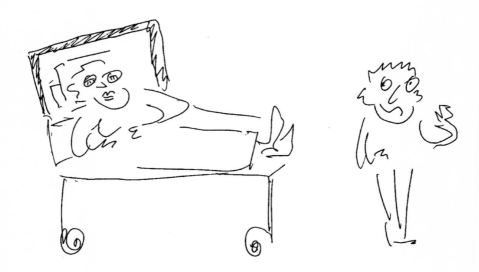

My wife, who is my rock, takes ill and is hospitalized with spinal meningitis.

Since I can't drive, due to my seizures, I am forced to hitch-hike down the mountain when I go to visit her in the hospital. This really pisses me off!! I feel like I am being punished even though it wasn't me that caused the accident by poor driving. The guys who hit me are probably back on the road and it was totally their fault!

Now my wife is being transferred to Vancouver because of serious complications and I have to fly down to be with her.

The whole idea of traveling to Vancouver by myself terrifies me! How will I find my way through the airport? How will I find the hospital? How will I find the apartment of the friend I will stay with? It all seems insurmountable!

I am traveling towards the edge of a cliff. My steps are brittle—limited to the little victories of finding the correct ticket wicket, baggage claim, and bus line. Once I am in Vancouver I discover that I can walk from my friend's apartment to the hospital. I walk the same way every day, almost in my previous day's footsteps! I am so afraid I will lose my way in the city. In the hospital I also travel with the same caution I use in the outside world so I won't get lost there.

Somehow I am aware that taking care of my wife is helping me find myself. I even dare to go to the beach and jog along the paths. I feel a little bit of confidence in myself. My wife's tests work out okay and she is scheduled to come home soon. The scare for her health is over.

Back home I am again at the dining table with my head in my hands. Over and over I tell my wife that I want to go back to California and find myself! There is a big hole in me and I hate everything. I have lost my spirit.

CHAPTER 9

WHAM BAM THANK YOU MAM

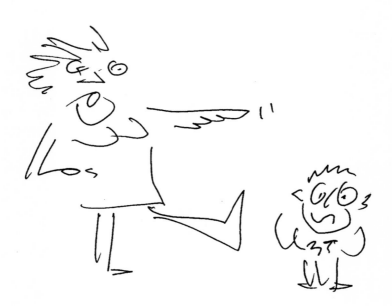

My wife who has troubles of her own is healthy enough to tell me: "Okay! Get out of here! Go find yourself in California!!" Even though we hardly have money to eat, she miraculously comes up with extra cash to send me, and my two oldest sons, to California by bus. This really frightens me because traveling by bus is slow, ugly and relies on maintaining a fairly good mood to survive the grueling conditions. I am hopelessly depressed and do not want to lay it on my boys. I am also greatly afraid of having a seizure in public as I still don't trust my drugs. Every time I feel weird, which is often, I think one is coming on.

In the Vancouver bus terminal, waiting between connections, I have a panic attack because I think I am starting to have a seizure. I start to tremble and my sons take me to a corner where they hug me until I feel secure enough to break down into tears. I wonder how this must feel to a couple of teenagers who used to look upon their father as a pillar of strength and the font of all wisdom. Mercifully the boys keep their thoughts to themselves and I steel myself for the trip.

The bus ride is pure torture. Nothing I can do, including reading and trying to enjoy the company of my sons can keep me from experiencing the grip of my depression. I have no idea of what this trip is supposed to accomplish. It is just a living hell of dirty plush seats and back of the bus washrooms that waft their sour odors. I try to curl up and disappear into sleep but it only seems to come half way. The boys have found seats of their own.

Bus stations along the way are terrifying and I feel like everyone is staring at me and aware of my misery. The boys buy me sandwiches and soft drinks and feed me like a helpless child. This is how I start my Vision Quest.

CHAPTER 10

TURNING POINT

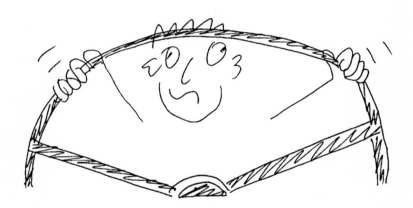

I am met at the small town bus station by my old friend and ex-land partner, who warmly welcomes me back to the old community. I don't remember telling him that I was coming down for a visit, but am really glad to see him.

He drives me up the mountain to his property and puts me up on the floor of an extra bedroom. Even though he is treating me with kindness, I find myself irritated and depressed because I sense him relating to me with old expectations. He just doesn't get it! I *can't* be my old self! I am snappy and finally blow up at him trying to explain what it feels like to

be so messed up. This friend senses my discomfort and backs off making the suggestion that I find other arrangements for a place to stay.

Another neighbor, somehow has the ability to understand my plight
and, hearing of my troubles, offers to put me up in his cabin for a couple of weeks. This happens to suit both of us well for his wife and children have gone on vacation, leaving him alone. The neighbor also
kindly lets me use his truck, which I used to drive often in the old days
when we shared it as a neighborhood vehicle. The truck has gotten very
funky since I last drove it and I am barely able to control it. I feel small
and weak in the torn and sagging seat wrestling with the large loose
steering wheel and am always afraid that I will drive it off the road. It
seems that I can hardly look over the hood in front of me. I wonder if its
owner knows how dangerous I am to the well being of his property. He
still must think that I am strong like I used to be in the old days when I
drove in extreme four-wheel drive conditions and had his complete
confidence. Again, I feel like a fraud.

I am using the truck to drive around the neighborhood to look at
vacant cabins and houses in the hope of finding a place to reestablish
residence in my old community. Each excursion is fraught with danger
as I lamely maneuver the old truck down narrow dirt roads and up
deeply rutted driveways, purposely left that way to keep the cops out.
This used to be my territory and I cringe at the thought of bringing my
family back to the substandard cabins and trailers, which I find haunted
with cobwebs and splitting apart. I don't believe I have the energy to set
up another homestead and doubt my ability to do so if I did. Seeing the
physical barriers to my dreams throws me further into depression about
this seeming impossibility of carving out any future for myself and my
family. I return to the cabin stunned and bummed.

My friend puts me to work helping him build the foundation for an
addition to his cabin. This proves to be a stroke of therapeutic genius
and the more I work, the better I feel. He treats me with great respect
and compliments me for my good work rather than tearing me down

for my mistakes, of which I feel there are many. I seem to think that I am worthless and keep bothering my benefactor for more compliments, which have become my lifeblood of support. I constantly receive his heartfelt thanks and feel like a fraud because I know I must have done a bad job.

I also find out that another neighbor, who is out of town and has a well built house on spectacular land, is considering selling his homestead and figure I should check it out because there's no telling how much money I may get from my pending law suit.

Once again I brave the funky truck and roar off up the mountain to see if the shoe fits.

The neighbor's house is beautiful and very classy. I can imagine my family living in it and walk around assigning bedrooms and placing furniture. I wonder how much he is considering asking for the place and hope that it will be within my reach. Still, I am aware that the asking price would probably use up most of my settlement and make it necessary to find a job in the community.

I decide to drive down to town and look for work. My hunt nets a possible job at a local garage as a grease monkey for minimum wage. Nothing else seems to be available in the community and I realize that I am much more limited in my skills than I was before I was injured. Minimum wage greasing cars will not net me enough to support my family and I go back up the mountain disheartened and seeing the dream to return to my old community slipping through my fingers. The final blow comes when I am told, by my friend, that he has just received a call from the neighbor who is asking an impossibly high amount of money for his classy house.

I am devastated but somehow hold on to a positive vision of the future deep within myself. It is now time for a walk in the woods.

BACK IN THE
SADDLE AGAIN

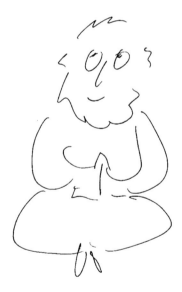

The neighbor's property borders our old land, which has a virgin fir forest crowned by a mountain top giant called "Momma Tree". The huge old fir is on the edge of a meadow and spreads its trunk-sized limbs out horizontally to take advantage of the open space around it. I used to climb into the tree and sit on these naturally elevated platforms to meditate when I was feeling I needed some connection with my higher self. I believed the spot had supernatural power for helping me sort myself out. Now may be a good time to sit in the tree.

I find familiar foot holds in the bark and amaze myself with unexpected physical strength as I once again ascend and settle into the body conforming mold of my old perch. My mind is full of anxiety and fear that I willfully try to push away so that I can experience the calm from which I hope to receive an inspiration that will save my life.

The noise in my head is mysteriously replaced by wind and the rustling of leaves from the forest below.

I can't explain how it happens, but somehow the idea to go back down the mountain and seek out the old superintendent of schools I used to work for to see if he has any work in his district for a school counselor pops into my mind. This superintendent knew me when I worked as a counselor/teacher for a small community alternative high school before I moved to Canada. He seemed to like my work with the kids and was especially appreciative of my ability to communicate well with both the alternative community and the more conservative school district. All my bells ring in accord with this idea and I really feel like I might be on to a real plan for the first time since my accident.

The superintendent remembers me and cordially invites me into his office. He listens to my story and request for work as a counselor in the district. However, he tells me that if he had employment, which he does not, he would require a specialized credential in "pupil personnel services" before he could hire me. He also tells me where to find programs which grant this credential—one at The University of California (which comes with a Masters of Social Work) and the other at San Francisco State University (which comes with a Masters of Counseling).

I am energized by this meeting and immediately decide to pursue entrance to the program at San Francisco State University because it is in counseling and is at my alma mater (I received a Bachelors of Fine Arts from S.F.S.U. twenty years ago and swore I would never go back to college).

It is less frightening to consider going to a school where I know the physical layout than to one I don't know as well. Less chance of getting lost.

Now I have a goal, which is congruent with my innermost hopes and dreams. I love working with teenagers and the job fits in with what a psychic told me I would do with my life. She said I would create music for children, which would help them heal. This idea has stuck with me as a guiding light throughout my depression though I had no idea how I could make it real since it appears that I have lost my ability to play music. Now I have a plan and surprisingly little fear in trying to make it happen. As much as I hate to leave the healing nature of living in the woods, I realize that I must travel by the horrid bus down to Berkeley to visit my mother and go over to San Francisco by train to check out the counseling department at the University. The prospect of all that public travel scares the hell out of me because I am never sure if or where I will have another seizure. I have decided to leave my sons in the country to give them a break from me and meet up with them later for the trip north to Canada. Somehow, after my message from the tree, I feel more confident and positive.

During my first visit to the University I feel as if I am in a fog, not quite knowing where my footsteps will land me. I also feel like I am being pulled along by a force that is greater than myself. Asking directions I find the counseling department and request the proper entry forms from the secretary who treats me in a motherly fashion, which makes me feel at home. It is my plan to take the forms back to Canada where I will fill them out and mail them after I discuss the logistics of the whole project with my wife. I know this path will mean a long separation from my family and I ask my mother if I can live with her in Berkeley for a couple of years. I do not intend to leave Canada permanently and make arrangements to borrow enough money from my mother to pay for my education until my lawsuit comes through. She is great and agrees to help me until I establish myself again as a man of means. I cannot wait to get home and get the ball rolling. I am very excited and have a great faith in the positive outcome of my future.

CHAPTER 12

TOON TIME

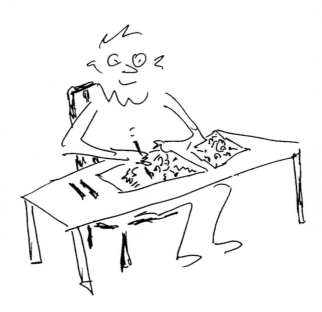

I arrive home with my new plans and find my wife extremely supportive, yet a bit apprehensive about a separation of the length I am proposing. She also feels, I imagine, validated for the wisdom of her choice to kick me out to find myself six weeks earlier. I send off the college application with high hopes. I notice, without shame, that I have played up the fact of my brain injury as a disability in hopes of positively influencing my chances for acceptance in a field (counseling), which I assume pays attention to politically correct affirmative action.

Either the time is right, or my hunch about being politically correct pays off, or it is *meant to happen*—I am accepted to the Masters Program in Counseling at San Francisco State University for the following year.

My neuropsychologist in Canada gives me a tentative blessing with the warning that I will have to work at least twice as hard in some areas as my non-injured colleagues. This does not discourage me, but rather makes me want to return to visit him some day on his level as a fellow professional.

The period between acceptance and leaving for school is sweet. It is like securing a job and not having to go to work until a later date. I can relax in the feeling that my future is secure.

It is during this time that I discover a dormant talent as a cartoonist. I have always drawn funny little creatures or doodles for home-made greeting cards throughout my life and now I have the leisure to expand my talent to visual puns which seem to assault me at every turn of the language. This could be a result of my brain injury for it seems that my verbal *gestalt* is always flipping back and forth. This phenomenon is not particularly uncomfortable, but serves to tickle my funny bone and inspires drawing after drawing, which I crank out by the hundreds.

A friend of mine, who has a small publishing company, is interested in putting a book together and I work with him to prepare a collection for publication. Part of me is still looking for identity and I fancy myself a Cartoonist, even though I know that I am on my way to University to become a counselor. This flutter of confusion does not bother me too much for I don't see any reason why one profession can't enhance the other. I am feeling a tremendous amount of freedom and fear uncontrollable euphoria—which scares me as much as depression.

CHAPTER 13

SHOE SHINE BOY

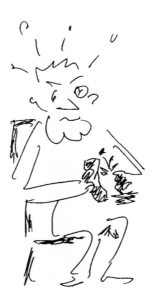

The time to leave for school arrives and I pull myself together because I know that I have been set on this path by a higher calling. Even though there are still doubts in my mind about *who I am* compared to *who I was*, I am beginning to depend on the current of my spiritual life, through the magical experiences in the tree in California, to help me define myself. It is with this new attitude that I begin my studies in University.

Life at my mother's is okay and I am settling into the rhythm of her one-woman (plus adult son) household. She dotes on me and is extremely supportive of my endeavors. I feel myself beginning to lose touch with my role as a husband and father in my own family. I wonder how this can be for it seemed so much a part of who I am. So I am actually *just going through the paces* of going to school and becoming a counselor. Part of me that is connected to my sense of worldliness is slipping away. I don't quite feel in control of who I am—or should I?

As I am struggling to take back my connection with the world of things I notice that my shoes are in need of a polish. This becomes a big project and I want to take back control of my life by buying some polish and doing it myself.

There is a shoemaker on a street near my mother's house. I ask him for some polish and he demonstrates how to apply it before he sells me the can. He reaches into the can and extracts the gooey brown substance with his bare fingers. Then he proceeds to smear it over the shoe and rub it in with his hand. I watch him closely so that I can do it correctly. Nowhere in my mind does it dawn on me to use a rag to apply the polish. I must do it just like this man whom I imagine eats breathes and sleeps shoe repair.

I go back to my mother's and proceed to polish my shoes exactly as I was shown. The result is good, as far as polishing the shoes goes, but I end up with brown stained hands which don't quite come clean no matter how I scrub them. I suppose I must learn how to polish my shoes in such a way that I am fit to go about in the world of commuters and counseling students and not look like I don't know what toilet paper is for!

School is okay, but I find myself at a real loss when it comes to typing papers. My left hand does not work well enough to type without making so many mistakes that it doesn't seem worth the try. I find a friend to type my first big assignment on her computer for me and marvel at her dexterity and ability to understand and use so sophisticated a tool. Her product is only good enough to use as a version to edit and I spend many painful hours arguing with my mother over the fine points of my writing which I don't want to lose as she chops my flowery verbiage down to Spartan sentences that tell the story better.

My mother figures that it is better if she types my papers herself so we can edit them directly from my hand written originals. What other student has their mother type papers for them at the age of 43? I must be the only geek whose arthritic old mother does this. I barely feel the thoughts are mine—the editing is so fierce!

Even though I still feel like a fraud, some of my teachers seem to be treating me like I am for real. Several of them have even taken a personal interest in me and seem to find value in my contributions in class. They even acknowledge that I am doing quite well in spite of my brain injury. They all know about it because I blab it to everyone I meet and write about it in my papers. When will I ever stop having to tell everyone that I was in a car wreck?

Life at my mother's is comfortable until we get into an argument about paying a phone bill. While she is making a fuss over sixty dollars and I whip out three twenties and slam them down on the table with rage and a few choice words. My mother rips up the bills and tries to stuff them in my mouth. I shake my head in wonder and toss her a roll of tape from a nearby drawer. After the bills have been reconstructed we have a good laugh and I realize that our life as house mates may have a time limit. It is a bittersweet moment.

CHAPTER 14

WHO'S ON FIRST

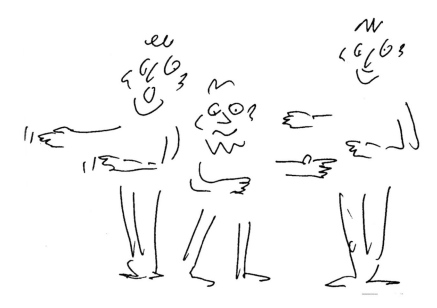

On my first trip home to Canada to visit my family for Christmas I do an astonishing and revealing thing at the airport. After leaving the plane and walking to the terminal, I plunge directly into the arms of my old-est son who is waiting with the family to greet me. This is not so remarkable in itself except that he is not the first member of the family in line to greet me. I have unwittingly passed by my third boy as if he

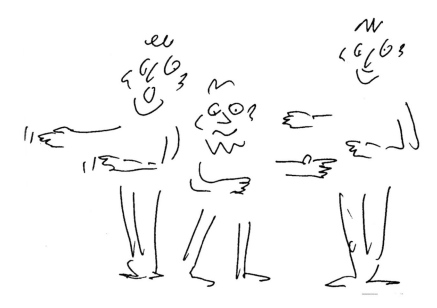

wasn't even there. He has to holler a loud "Dad!" to get my attention. I am flustered and slowly realize that it may not completely be my fault that I do not recognize him. During the four months I have been at school he has undergone tremendous changes of puberty and is all but a stranger with his great new height and oily complexion. I still have enough presence of mind to imagine how he must feel to have me pass him by without any recognition at all. He is my beloved child and I have been away while he has grown up. This strikes me as a tragedy and I tell my wife about it in the car.

She does not take more than a minute to state the obvious—We need to live together as a family or the kids will lose touch with me as their father during these times of dramatic growth in their life. We must all go to Berkeley and live in my mother's house until I finish school and we can move back to Canada.

We decide to pack up during the summer, rent the house, and move the family to California for the fall semester. This plan requires an awesome amount of organization: building storerooms in the barn, mothballing the truck, putting the house in shipshape order, finding renters, and helping to send our two older sons off to college for their first term. My lawsuit has come in so we have some money to operate with, which makes it easier to manifest the plans—but does not diminish the tremendous anxiety I feel as I go through the motions of preparing for the move to Berkeley. Nothing seems easy to me anymore in the world of organizing stuff but I know it is worth it to be with my family. I may have lost an image of myself as a competent person somewhere along the line—but not my love for my wife and kids.

THEY SAID IT COULDN'T BE DONE

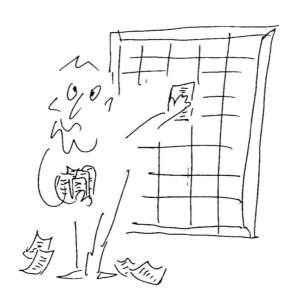

My mother takes us into her home with graciousness and an imaginary line down the middle of the refrigerator so that we don't mix our food with hers. We set up camp in the basement and share the use of the kitchen upstairs, which contains cooking facilities and the sub-divided refrigerator.

My wife has some choice words about my mother, which she saves for walks around the neighborhood. I try to point out both sides of whatever it is she is upset about and catch hell for defending my mother over her. This, I believe, is some age-old trap for husbands to fall into. I try to be nice in the vain hopes of winning favors and somehow don't feel completely like a fraud. I am definitely capable of making *real* mistakes in the family circus. The kids attend school in my old elementary and junior high schools. Nothing has changed much except the buildings are dilapidated and they have bussed in gobs of minorities which creates a racial balance in the schools that simply would not have been believed possible in my day. My wife becomes a parent volunteer in the elementary school and I land a practicum as a school counselor the junior high.

My supervising counselor, who reminds me of a childhood friend that I didn't like, is terribly efficient and treats me as if I am just a bit slow—which I may be after all. I love the kids and the funky ambience of the school. Most of the staff treats me with genuine warmth and I am told that I have the right tone of voice to become a great counselor. I have landed in heaven and am even sort of thankful that I had my accident and had to go back to school.

One day the supervisor gives me the task of putting notices in the teachers' boxes. She tells me that it shouldn't take long because the boxes are in alphabetical order. I go out in the hall and am dismayed to find that the placement of the boxes does not resemble alphabetical order at all as I study them from left to right. Completely baffled, I start to deposit the notices one by one to each teacher's individual box. This takes an agonizingly long time and I begin to realize that I have been out in the hall for about half an hour. The supervisor eventually comes out to hurry me up and seems a bit frustrated when she has to explain that the boxes are alphabetically ordered in rows from top to bottom. Why didn't I think of that? I feel really stupid and unworthy of my position as a student school counselor. Upon later reflection I realize that this is what the neuropsychologist was talking about when he said that I would have trouble going back to school! It is the same difficulty I experienced when the tests he gave me shifted criteria and required me to exercise the part of my brain that dealt creatively with anomalies. I understood the concept when the psychologist explained my low scores in the ability to change action plans. I could not foresee what difficulties this deficiency might create in my life. This is probably why I have so much trouble figuring out what to do at intersections and when the rules of the road are altered by the directions of hand held signs which demand me to change my sequential processing on the spot.

My school work is going well and I can see the light at the end of the tunnel. We live for the summers and eagerly look forward to the yearly return to our home in Canada. As much as I really hate the place for its being the site of my horrible accident and the deterioration of my wife's health, I love it for being my home and the future it promises in the reestablishment of myself as the working head of my family.

THEY GOT ME WHILE I'M DOWN

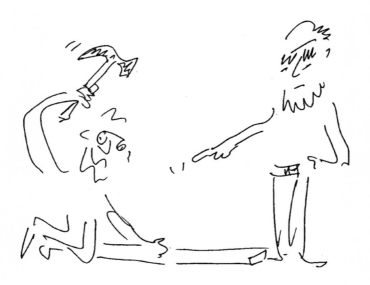

Summers are strange with associations that blur my reality and make me feel that I am not quite really here in my own house with the trappings of my manhood and memories of my competence. We have it set up so that the renters are out for the summer and we have our scene back pretty much as it was—except that I have lots of time to pretend that I am a real guy.

Somehow I have landed a job helping some friends build an office building downtown. I hope to make enough money to buy myself a new bicycle. My boss is an old man who fancies himself sort of a spiritual teacher. He is a real jerk and has a group of followers who think the sun rises and sets on him. I have befriended some of these followers in the hopes of living within a community and reestablishing myself as an important and respected person. These new friends treat me like I am stupid and I never feel like I belong no matter how much they pretend to like me. Their guru, the old carpenter, stalks me pointing out my physical clumsiness and intellectual ineptitude to the eternal delight of his disciples. The members of this group hang on his every word and never seem to take me seriously. I hate them and can't wait to get free even though there must be some pearls of wisdom to be gleaned from their trip. It's just that the pearls are layered with pain and don't make sense until later. I suppose, to carry the metaphor further, the old guru is like a grain of sand and agitates me to create pearls of my own. For this I am thankful but I won't ever forget his awesome ignorance.

On the job the he tells me, as I am struggling in slow motion to unravel a deep mystery of spatial perception buried in the proper placement of a 2X4, "I'd rather be 74 years old like me, than 44 and slow like you!" I reply, with sudden heat, "You want to know why I'm so slow? It's because I have a brain injury and it takes me more time to figure out where things go!" He stops to inform me that I have to "try and be stronger than my handicap"—all it takes is "will" or some damn word he has stolen and is passing on to his closest followers with particular definition. Obviously I am left out of the loop. I hate the man tremendously and bite my tongue when a woman on the job, who is one of his most devoted followers, tells me with wide eyes: "He must really care for you or he wouldn't take the time to correct you." Even though I am livid, I reply that she must be right and I really am lucky. What a wimp! I can't even tell it like it is to these brain washed idiots. I have sunk that low. This makes me more upset than the old man's abuse. I have lost my ability to stand up for myself as an individual. And I am training to be a counselor! It's not really my fault. They got me while I'm down.

Aside from our relationships with the carpenter's cult, we have few friends left in Canada. Going back to California in the fall is a disjointing experience for it takes us away from whatever sense of home we have left after over 25 years of building a scene. This is sad to me and I blame my car accident for it. Property and possessions are left set up like a stage set in Canada waiting for the completion of my education before I can participate as an active member in my life. I still feel more real as a student but rely on the life I have put on hold for my credibility in the world. My self-image is as confused as ever.

In spite of the middle class implications, I have decided, at my wife's urging, to buy a brand new car. The old station wagon, which we ended up with after trading in the silver *Jeep* to pay off some debts, is needing more and more repairs. Going to the car dealers with money from the lawsuit in our pockets is a strange experience. I feel my values changing without me.

We are wined and dined by salesmen who treat us like people of property and I let myself be swept up in the game even though I know I have no future financial stability. The salesmen don't see this and buy my story of being able to make payments on fancy trucks and vans without me even having a job. They must be hungry and don't understand the financial peril they are putting themselves in.

After all is said and done we end up with a posh four-wheel drive van that is completely foreign to my country boy sensibilities. I am terrified with the responsibility of owning such a perfect new thing and neurotically spend extra money on having my investment rust proofed. I have become the quintessential white man consumer but have no idea of how to support myself in the workaday-rat race-professional-world. The attempt to find myself in becoming a professional counselor is becoming confused with my image of its trappings. I feel like I am on a runaway freight train of material acquisition.

CHAPTER 17

AXE MURDERER

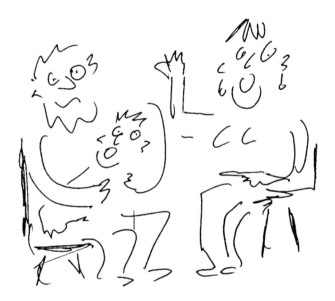

Going back to Berkeley in the fall to live at my mother's and go to school, catapults me into my student life. Now I am a student with a fancy car that has British Columbia plates and lights that stay on all the time to meet Canadian safety requirements. California drivers are forever honking their horns and yelling "Your lights are on!" They are *so* helpful it drives me nuts.

I go to school like I am going to a job and yearn for the day my life can begin again. I tell my fellow students how wonderful it is in my Canadian hometown and how I am going back after graduation to live a great life. I almost believe it myself and only have to look at the shiny new van parked outside my mother's house to reinforce the dream. I feel pretty weird and wonder about what I am becoming.

My last year at school finds me in a practicum at my old high school, which is huge, with 3,000 students, and intriguing because of its great diversity. I must be getting better because even though the school is much more complex than my last placement at the junior high, I am less confused and more able to make my way around. The junior high has offered me a real part-time job which helps with our living expenses. I am able to go back and forth between job, practicum placement, and classes in San Francisco with a facility I only dreamed of a short time ago.

Though I seem to operate better in worldly matters, I still don't feel like myself. I am experiencing distinct uneasiness in an advanced group therapy class. Once again I don't recognize myself in a manner which is comfortable with what I remember as myself-image. Does one remember a self-image or is it something that is not supposed to be separate and distinguishable at all?—even as a memory? I am finally able to experience the illusion of my separation with enough perspective to feel myself coming into focus.

Some things have changed on a fundamental level within my personality. I have become less agreeable. This surfaces in a group therapy class which is run like an actual therapy group. I find myself challenging the professor almost like a teenager challenging his father. The rest of the group seems phony and whiny to me and I feel like a misfit around their "we-are-a-one-big-happy-family-let's-support-one-another" attitude. No one seems genuine and I experience myself standing alone in the group when I am supposed to be all "nicey-nicey-goody-goody-feel-good" during the sessions. I hate what I perceive as the group's phoniness and hate myself as well for not participating in the artificially induced community of my fellow students. I feel out of the loop again. When will I ever come back to myself?—or maybe this slightly crusty guy *is* myself. Could I ever grow to like him? This is a very unsettling but hopeful question. Maybe I am experiencing the emergence of a new me? I suppose there must be some strange and unknown dimensions to be explored if I ever hope to cut through this feeling of separation and experience a sense of unity within myself.

The therapy class/group is having a party at the professor/therapist's house. One woman in the group, whose infant son has just undergone heart surgery, wins the undying support and sympathy of the whole group. I like her well enough but am a little peeved with the group for fawning over her so much. Everyone is *so* supportive it makes me sick. I feel like an outsider because I do not feel about her what I perceive my colleagues to be feeling. *I am too busy feeling that way about myself.* She brings her baby to the gathering and passes him around the table for all to hold. The baby fusses and screams in my arms and I imagine that his response to being in contact with me has revealed me for the unsympa-thetic bastard that I seem to have become. This is very unsettling because I used to think of myself as a 100 percent nice guy. The mother makes me feel better by saying that the baby sometimes carries on uncontrollably. I feel alone because I was the only person in whose arms the baby cried. All the others look at me as if I am an axe murderer. I hate them and feel like an outsider when I think I am supposed to be feeling warm and fuzzy. Talk about uncomfortable! What is happening to me?

While I am in Berkeley one of my friends from the carpenter's cult, who is a registered psychologist, sends me application forms to a pro-fessional counseling association in British Columbia. He is offering me a leg up into the professional community and suggests that I look into renting office space in the up-scale downtown building he has just erected. I guess he is looking for renters to help pay for it. This is the same building I worked on during the summer and I know it is a classy joint. I struggle with the forms and finally, after an agonizingly long time, feel comfortable enough to mail them to Canada. Just like *it's meant to be,* I am accepted into the "British Columbia Association of Clinical Counselors". It seems my place in the professional community is set up and I look forward to my return to the world of work with even more confidence.

School has been an exciting adventure but I am not quite sure how, or if, it has transformed me as I hoped it would. The toughest part of the program was making sure I had all the forms turned in on time so the bureaucracy would graduate me. I don't know how it has come to be, but I am a *Master of Science* in Counseling. This amazes me and confuses me even more because it is a degree of expertise that I did not aspire to as my old self. I hardly know what it means and am thankful to my mother for her graduation gift of a new sport coat that reflects the image of what a "professional" is supposed to look like.

CHAPTER 18

CLOTHES MAKE THE MAN

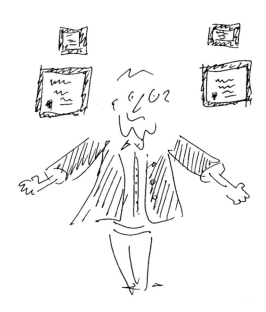

I have all the trappings: office, degree, sport coat, association member-
ship, fancy car, and private practice. My Canadian friends treat me with
the respect accorded my professional station and somehow this feels

horribly hollow. I have achieved my goal but still feel that I don't know who I am.

The only people I feel an affinity for are my clients, but I am told, by colleagues that it is unethical to feel this way. I can't imagine why they say that and continue to unwittingly blur what they perceive as professional boundaries. Once again Carl Jung comes to my rescue with a quote that says something like: "The therapist who does not allow himself to become friends with his clients is missing the whole purpose of the therapeutic relationship." This quote speaks a deep truth to me and I slip one notch closer to myself. It seems the path to experiencing unity may lie in the ability to put myself in contact with what I perceive as the truth. This seems an awesome task and sometimes I wish I were a simpler man.

CHAPTER 19

GOOD GRIEF

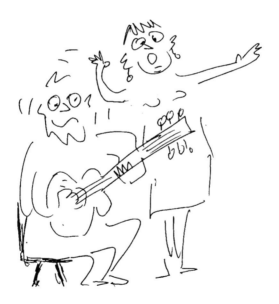

The wife of the psychologist down the hall is rehearsing a song for her church with a colleague in an adjoining office. The door is open and I can hear the poor guy struggling to accompany her. She has a pretty voice but sings so haltingly that she cannot lead the song. The poor accompanist flounders and inspires my deepest sympathy. Listening, I am lulled into a false sense of competency and think to myself that I could do better for I used to be a first class accompanist before my accident and, as such, could draw out the shyest singer.

Emboldened, I ask my friend if I might try the guitar. He hands me the instrument and I earnestly try to get in the groove. Nothing happens. I twang out a couple of chords, but the fluidity and skill I so hoped for do not come. I feel a great let down deep in my body and hand back the guitar. The psychologist's wife, who is a disciple of the carpenter guru, tells me to try to overcome it with my will. All I have to do is "try". This enrages me and I start to yell at her that she does not know what it is like to be brain injured. Then I stomp out of the room and slam the door between our offices.

After my explosion, I am sitting in one of my counseling easy chairs trying to breathe deeply and process what has just happened in the other room. Again I feel like an unbalanced and troublesome person—not at all how I pictured myself before my injury. This assessment of myself does not help me and pushes me farther back into my confusion. The old "before-and-after" trick is losing its effectiveness. This means that there must be something else to learn. Here I am sitting in this chair wearing this damn sport coat. The lesson is so close I can taste it. Day after day I sit in this very spot helping clients deal with their lives. Then it hits me! The psychologist's wife is not a stupid bitch, but a trigger for my grief about not being able to play the guitar. I have dumped it on her in the form of anger in response to her genuine attempt to help me. I must go tell her it is not her I am angry at. I hope I haven't hurt her feelings too badly.

She accepts my apology graciously and goes back to her feeble singing. My buddy with the guitar comes into my office later to see how I am doing. He is really distressed and has worried about me due to the emotional intensity I displayed in his office. His heart is in the right place but I don't think even he understands what I am going through. Nobody does. I wonder what it would feel like to find someone who really knows? That would be so sweet.

The same friend who plays guitar in the office next door also turns me on to the grieving process. He does this in a very informal and simple way by explaining that when we lose something, anything, we cycle through ourselves six emotions in a random order until the emotions fade and we don't need to do it anymore. These emotions are: anger, sadness, shock or numbness, denial, guilt, and fear. This information stuns me because they didn't mention anything about grief in counseling school. It sounds really important and I want to learn a whole lot more about it. There must be a textbook or a course somewhere that I could get my hands on. My buddy next door seems pretty knowledgeable on the subject and I pump him for all he knows. What I get is a sense that this is something that I should be paying close attention to for the good of my clients—and myself. I learn that the grieving process has no linear pattern and that one phase of emotion does not always follow another. The emotion that is needed for healing shows up on its own in an organic fashion much like hormones are released to bring about the race of proper blood cells to an injured part of the body. This suits me fine for I would rather trust my healing process to my own internal healer than to the manifestation of carefully worked out intellectual schemes based on statistics. I am learning to trust my own process of healing to provide me with the best results—even though I am not so sure of who I am. I feel I am in for a great journey of self-discovery now that I am acknowledging the fact that my emotional responses are valid. I am so excited that I reach down inside myself and come up with a personal metaphor to explain the phenomenon of the grieving process.

When I was a little boy roaming the acorn ridden reaches of my Thousand Oaks neighborhood canyon backyard in Berkeley, I was amazed by the multitude of acorns left on the ground by the prickly leafed trees. These acorns, I figured, provided food for the canyon's original human inhabitants when ground up into a mash and mixed with water. I found ample evidence of this activity in the primitive stone mortars and pestles unearthed by my excavations for childhood forts in the root-ridden hillsides. I also marveled at hollows carved into the tops of creek side channel stones, which gave more evidence to my theory that the natives pounded their acorns directly beside the creek so they could mix them with water.

I was so excited about my discovery that I told it to everyone I thought would be impressed—or whom I thought I could impress. One such person was a neighbor who was a professor at the University. He burst my bubble of deduction by informing me that I had missed a crucial step in the process of hunter-gathering. This was the sad fact that the glorious yellow/orange colored acorns were poisonous if processed and eaten directly after they were harvested. They had to be put into a basket and allowed to soak in the creek so the running water could pass through them and leach the poison out over a rather long period of time like several months or weeks, I don't remember which.

To me the grieving process is like the acorns in the basket cycling the loss in the stream of healing emotion until it is painless enough that we can go on living. The pain is never really totally gone and we are never like we were before we experienced it but we are eventually healed enough so that we can go on with our lives.

This metaphor is very helpful to me as I live my life in the *basket of my grief* and work to acknowledge the *stream of my emotions.* I can't figure out why they didn't teach me this in counseling school. Still it is revelations like this which spark my creativity and bring me closer to becoming myself. Client after client allows me to witness the rightness of my understanding and give me the reflection that I am in the right place in my life. I wonder if I have lost myself in my profession.

This is not a vain wonderment for me because of the keen distinction I am making between the process of my creativity, which I resonate with, and the product of my professionalism, which I perceive the world is defining me by. Interestingly enough I am finding more identity and material for my self-image as a *creator* than as a professional counselor. My community does not reflect this and I am increasingly unhappy with my status as a middle-class professional. I want to live a life that is in keeping with my emerging self-image. I have only one friend among my peers, outside of my wife, who reflects this new self-image and he, in turn, has only one friend—me. We are a club of two and, aside from the time we spend validating each other's uniqueness, I am lonely and feel invisible to, and resentful of, the rest of my friends and acquaintances. Everyone knows me as a local therapist and treats me with deference. I suppose I should be delighted with my new station in life but it feels like a hollow victory.

The lawyer told me, way back when, that our goal was to get enough from the lawsuit to put me *back the way I was.* I naively accepted this, not understanding that, no matter how successfully I am able to return to functional life in the world, *I can never feel exactly like the person I was before my injury.* Maybe my folly is that I took the lawyer literally and had no real experience with brain injuries and consciousness of the grieving process.

Who is this new guy I am becoming? Is he different or the same? Are the differences only the fact that irrelevant parts were burnt off by the trauma of becoming. Was the old built upon illusions, or is something vital missing from me? These questions plague me, and may be part of the new me.

Is this the natural result of brain injury? Am I destined to live the rest of my life always not quite being sure? Is this a good thing? I wonder if a certain tentativeness is not bad? Sometimes being too cocksure tends to blind me to the reality of a more fluid self. My life seems a flower waiting to unfold.

ODE TO JOY

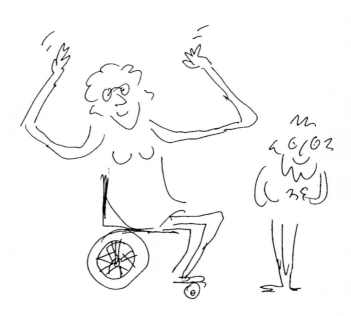

My wife has befriended an old disabled woman who is a profound artist and philosopher. She has told this woman that I am both an artist and musician. This is not untrue and does not clash with whatever image of myself as a creative being I have managed to keep alive through my ordeal. My wife tells me the old woman wants to meet me and show me a work of art that was inspired by Beethoven's Ninth Symphony because

I am both musical and visual. I am intrigued and look forward with great joy to meet and be taken into the creative confidence of an artist whose work I have seen and admired.

I am led into the living room of a beautiful old house and greeted with deep respect and interest. I am not quite sure how to respond to being treated as an equal by someone I think is so great. I cannot remember this happening to me since my accident and a part of me I have forgotten, but has always been there, begins to flutter awake from a seeming lifetime of sleep.

The old woman brings my attention to an album, which displays a pieced together photograph of an awesome painting that stretches across the page in bursts of color and shape that somehow speak directly to my soul. I am informed that the original work is stored in a museum in Alberta. It, along with some forty–five others in a remark-able series of her life's work, is awaiting a showing that is worthy of its stature. The fate of this work pales in my mind as she sets up an old per-sons' version of a ghetto blaster (mono, with only one speaker) and clicks in a tape of the first movement of the *Ninth.*

As strains of music begin to crackle from the feeble speaker, her overly long arthritic old arms begin to wave in the air and dance between photograph and music. I wonder why she is satisfied with such a sub-standard tape player before I am transfixed by the experi-ence of a subtle renaissance of electrochemical connection. Aside from my cartooning and the experience of reading Jung's autobiography, this feeling is the first real inkling of the *muse* that I have been aware of since my head injury. In an instant I feel my artistry and professional training (counseling) melding together to illuminate the fact that *human resonance with certain shapes promotes psychological health.* This flashes into my theoretical mind as a potential tool, which I can even-tually use with clients.

I rush back to my counseling practice with a creative impetuousness that I am learning to recognize as a hallmark of my post-injury mode of operating. This impetuousness seems to serve me well in my rapidly executed cartoons but I find I have to use lots of paper until I get it right. I wonder how many clients I will confuse with my wild ideas before I get it right?

CHAPTER 21

SHAPES ALIVE

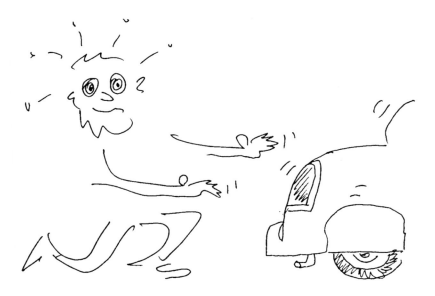

I am inundated with creativity and run around seeing healing shapes in everything. I desperately want to try my theory out on clients and don't wait for it to be lab tested. I start in right away asking people, what natural settings they prefer, what favorite objects make them feel good, what type of car they drive, (and what part of the car makes them feel good when they look at or touch it?). I am like a crazy man and the clients either indulge me or find it helpful—even if it is a bit far out. My wife encourages me and we spend most of the road time on our next trip to California discussing our feelings about the shapes of cars we pass on the highway. We really get into it. I finally feel like I have a purpose—or we have gone completely nuts. I haven't felt this alive since I was building Community Centers in California!

CHAPTER 22

FOOLSCAP

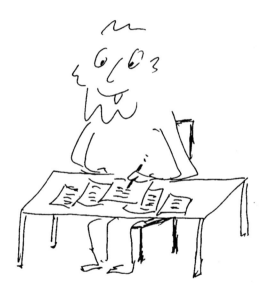

Our California vacation is remarkable for bringing encouragement, from a professor I knew in school, to write up my Shape Therapy ideas into an academic paper. She urges me to prepare it for submission to an international counseling conference in Vancouver the following year. I am inspired by the suggestion and a bit unsure of myself because of the responsibility to write and *type* the required 5,000 words.

We return home and I dig into yet another year of full time counseling for the province-wide employee assistance program I have worked for over the last two years. I like the counseling well enough but can't shake the feeling that I am an impostor. The regional director, who hired me, seems to be overly critical as I have received mixed reviews on my client evaluation sheets. This process pisses me off because the evaluations, which are anonymous to keep client confidentiality intact, are sometimes very strong in their criticism or praise of my counseling. I would be very grateful to know which of my clients are helped or turned off by the specific techniques I am employing in their therapy. This process makes me feel vulnerable to the small-mindedness of my boss who's quest, as I perceive it, is to show me that I am not free as long as I work for him.

There is, however, one particular client who has a major breakthrough using my Shape Therapy. He is only one of several I have tried my theory on and as such is not really a great statistical indicator of its success. This does not slow me down in the slightest, but inspires me to leap forward in the advanced application of my theoretical ideas. I wonder if I am being professionally irresponsible because of the lack of science but brush the thought aside in favor of my penchant for creative impetuosity. Why do I feel so urgent about everything?

When I go back to the drawing board of my theoretical exploration, I find myself inspired to write my offering to the upcoming conference and blithely decide to use my one and only great success as the case history for my paper. Five thousand words seems daunting for I have, more and more, come to think of myself as a man of few words. I am also wondering how I will get the damn thing typed if I can manage to produce that much verbiage.

Surprisingly the paper flows out of me easily in handwritten form. I crank out 50 plus pages of pencil-laden foolscap and give it to a colleague, who moonlights as an English instructor at a local college, to edit for me. She returns my work with some constructive criticism and encourages me by taking the time to ask me more about my theory as she is thinking of using some of the therapeutic tools from the paper in her own practice. I am greatly encouraged by this and pass the corrected manuscript on to my daughter-in-law to type for me. When she returns it I can send it in to the conference selection committee. I am sending in my entry with the same mixture of confidence and terror that I felt when I applied for graduate school.

Again, *just as it is meant to be,* I am accepted as a presenter at the conference and am asked to send a copy of my paper to be published in the conference journal. I feel like both a million bucks and an impostor at one and the same time. How has this happened to me? I never aspired to become an academic but here it is, and it seems to be on my own terms. The momentum of my paper is propelled by my newfound impetuous creativity. My paranoia of being discovered as a scientific fraud returns. What will they say at the conference when they discover that I have never done this before?

I go about proving myself an impostor by passing the paper around to certain unimaginative people, including my boss, whom I know just won't get what I am talking about. They don't. This fuels my uneasiness and contributes to putting me more and more on edge as the date for the conference nears.

CHAPTER 23

PHOENIX

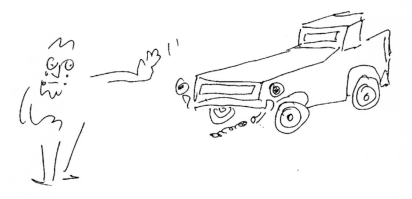

I have finally come to grips, after some persuasion from my wife, with the fact that I must sell my beloved old army truck to raise enough money to go to Vancouver for the upcoming conference. We decide to build our summer vacation around the conference and I secretly wonder if I will be fit company to travel with because I have become so anxious about exposing myself to my colleagues. I don't tell anyone about my fears and go numbly, like a heartless robot, through the motions of selling the truck. I know that I will have re-occurring dreams about the truck because I am dimly aware that it is a symbol for some deeply rooted part of my old self-image as a back-to-the-land self-sufficient householder. I am also somewhat reconciled to the creation of a myth that a new life is rising out of the ashes of my old one, and have decided to let the truck go, because it makes sense that it might have been consumed in that sacred fire.

After I organize time off from work, we make our travel plans and set off on the next transformation of our life together. I am incredibly uptight and spend most of my time on the road raging at my wife and son. Somewhere in myself I have to admit that my behavior is the cause of this horrible tension in the car, although I would love to blame it on the other members of my family. Once again the message is clear that we must change our life or wither. We don't know how our new life will present itself—only that this trip is the true path to find it. I have a deep sense of trust, within the tempest of my fear, that we will find our way.

CHAPTER 24

DIRECTIONAL SIGNAL

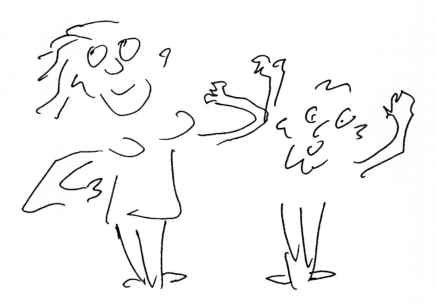

Our first stop is in Vancouver for me to attend my conference. I am in a terrible state. We are staying at the parents of my second son's wife for a day before and after the conference, which is to be held at a big hotel downtown and will last two days. After the conference we plan to explore Vancouver Island and do some camping. My son's parents-in-law are very distant emotionally and seem to resent our being there. I foist my paper on the step-mother, who is a health professional, and am not surprised when she doesn't understand it. Her response fires up my panic around being discovered as a fraud at the conference and I spend my time at her house in a brittle forest of anxiety. I also use my spare time to acquaint myself with Vancouver's public transportation and make a couple of trial runs from the condo to the hotel downtown so I don't get lost on my way to the all important conference and arrive late for registration.

I try to contain my fear and go through the motions of being reasonable company to my wife and son who are acting like saints in their attempts to help me keep calm.

One evening, as I am walking in a local park with my wife, she pauses to inform me that she has just had a vision. My wife's visions have sort of acted as signposts in the unfolding of our life together and I have come to trust and welcome them as indications that we are on the right track. Nothing could make me feel better. The vision is of *mist revealing a sculpted rock formation reaching into the sea with trees and grass leading down to the water.* It is not so much the physical description of the scene that impresses her, but the *profound feeling of peace and well being that accompanies it—and the absolute conviction that such a place or state of mind exists within our future.* I am now sure, for the first time since my accident, that we will once again find harmony in our lives and feel my anxiety retreat in the path of my faith. I feel more at ease about the conference because I know it is not all-important but just another step in becoming myself again.

The next morning finds me in freshly ironed clothes, ready to brave the Sky Train. I notice with bemusement, as I pass by the front door, my son's father-in-law's shoes that he wears to his work as a heavy duty mechanic, are exactly the same as those I have chosen for the conference rooms of academia—only his look like they have been soaked in engine oil. Oh Well, I never was much of a clothes horse—except in the days when I wore knee high Vibram soled boots and embroidered hippie badges on my jean jacket. Then, I used to strut in armor. Now, I feel much more exposed and enter the lobby of the great hotel on soft soles.

What will they think of my theory? I am amazed that my name is actually on the list of presenters and gratefully accept my conference package and nametag from a table by the elevators. I am scheduled to give my presentation the morning of the second day. Until then I will attend the "welcome" and sessions on subjects of interest to me.

Before my presentation rolls around I have met many who treat me with a respect as a colleague and that is encouraging. I can hardly believe that all these highly educated people in my field are treating me like an equal! Maybe I am a *real* professional after all. My fears seem to be melting away in the presence of so much acceptance. I go back to the in-laws with less tension and relate more peacefully with my family.

The next day my presentation goes pretty well and I sense a real interest in my work. These people understand what I am up to! I begin to feel truly validated though I suspect that the conference is an artificial mutual admiration society. God! This lack of self-confidence must be really deep to remain in the presence of so much validation! Still, I feel great after my presentation and begin to accept the genuine interest some of the conference members are showing in me and my work. Where will it all lead? I never would have believed I could get so far in the world—even *before* my accident! Still I am not quite so sure that this reflection, positive though it is, is not just one sparkling piece of the mirror of my shattered self-image. I have been tricked by not so positive reflections in my attempts to piece myself together as a whole person. I never asked these questions before my brain injury. *Maybe I am closer to myself than I appear*—and I will never *get it* until I stop trying to experience so self-consciously.

One would think that I would now be able to relax and enjoy the rest of my vacation camping with my family—but it is not so. The trip gets worse and worse as I feel the pressure to rebuild my life up to the standard of the glorious conference. This life seems to require going back to school to obtain a Ph.D. so that I can legitimately call myself an academic (*Doctor Mogerman I presume?*). My wife thinks this is the route to go and leans on me to press some contacts with the University of Victoria that I made at the conference. I say "yeah, yeah" and hope it will get her off my back. All I really want to do is quit my uptight job and get the hell out of the Okanagan Valley, which I have really come to hate.

We go to the ocean and I walk the beaches in a daze while trying to center myself on my wife's vision and the belief that all this suffering will end some day when I find the right place in the world, or within myself, and stop thinking about it.

After a miserable stay in a coastal campground, we drive across Vancouver Island to visit a couple of islands in the Georgia Strait which we heard were good places for artists to live. While poking around an island community center I suddenly get the feeling that *this is where I belong!* It is not University, but Community that I yearn for. The pieces of my shattered mirror seem to coalesce in one brief moment and I feel like I could throw away my artificial professional life, along with my academic aspirations, and move to these islands. My family looks at me with fear because they know I will do this. I don't know it yet, but the coastline around these islands closely meets the physical requirements of my wife's vision. Not knowing, or caring, how long it will take to manifest my dream we return home with the plan for me to apply to a Ph.D. program. Nobody says anything about my island epiphany. Some things are best left to work themselves out.

CHAPTER 25

ENGAGEMENT RING

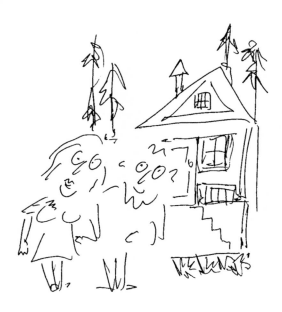

At my wife's urging I apply to a Ph.D. program and receive some encouragement from a professor I met at the conference. He invites me to Victoria to discuss the matter in his office at the University. We stay with one of my sons in his apartment on the University campus grounds. I feel depressed and experience actual physical pain in my lower chest, which proves to be an ulcer. I know that I don't want to go

74

back to school but keep up a front for my wife. My heart is in the Gulf Islands and I secretly pray that I won't be accepted into the Ph.D. program even though it will disappoint my wife. My interview with the professor confirms my feelings of antipathy towards academic research and makes me realize that I would be setting myself up for battles with the University in which I would probably be ultimately squashed. We return to the Okanagan and I still go about making application to the Ph.D. program. I must be nuts or I am afraid to get off my ass and follow my heart.

Luckily, the University turns down the application and I can legitimately say to my wife that I sincerely tried to get back into school. What we both seem to tacitly accept is that I only tried to gain entrance to *one* graduate school and its rejection was cause enough to quit the chase.

We immediately put our house up for sale and I enjoy a glorious state of knowing that I am going to quit my job. Even though I believe it is the right thing to do, I have great fears about selling out and moving to a new area without work. I literally jump off the mattress in my bed at night in fear of the unknown and mourn the impending loss of my middle class security.

The house takes several months to sell and during that time we get the name of a Gulf Islands realtor who sends us his local listings. Nights, we sit around the table together mooning over places that look interesting to us. The next thing to do is to take another trip to the islands and explore some of the properties that have caught our fancy in the listings. This will be our second trip to the islands and we go with a more conscious eye towards discovering any manifestation of my wife's vision that might lead us to the land of our fulfillment.

I have built up some vacation time and it is not hard to snatch a couple of days off work. There is much more purpose to this trip and I feel in better spirits—even excited with the prospect of a future. I have not felt this way in a long time because I couldn't imagine enough of myself to project into the future. The stay at my son's house in Victoria is more tolerable and I am less grumpy and depressed than I have been on previous visits. The closer we get to the islands, the more focused I feel. It seems strange that I haven't been able to do what I really want to do with my life since the drunks hit me. I have only been able to do what I have had to do to survive and rehabilitate myself. This is not to say that the schooling and visions that helped me along the way are not valid experiences. It's just that I felt I was not experiencing life as a complete person.

We meet the realtor, who is a nice guy, and he takes us on a house tour around two islands in the Strait of Georgia. We choose to focus our search on the inner of the two because it looks closer to my wife's vision and closer to Vancouver Island, should I find work there.

During the tour we are shown a listing that is probably way out of our reach financially. It inspires us to dream about working together to create a center for the arts and healing on the property. We have been together far too long to put much stock in the literal unfolding of such dreams and recognize that we are finally engaging in the process of projecting our lives together after years of fearful retreat due to our tragedies.

On the drive back to our son's in Victoria, we fill the time with euphoric embellishments of our future dreams. It all seems very real and it feels great. I feel that a bubble has burst and I can finally be truly light hearted again.

CHAPTER 26

GROUND ZERO

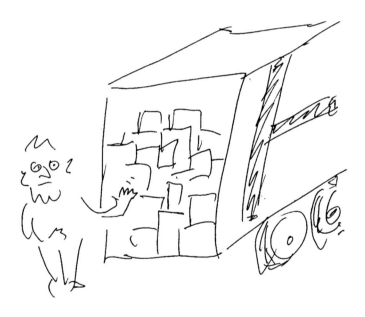

Arriving home, we take out a big loan against the sale of the house and kick into high gear to fix up the place and make it irresistible to prospective buyers. I still jump in my bed at the thought of what will happen if my hopes and dreams for a new life on the island don't work out. What if I don't find work? What if someone gets sick? Why am I leaving all this security? These bouts of fear last for only about an hour in the early mornings and the rest of my days are spent in a charge of creative energy that I put into my counseling, and a new theory that springs on me while I am working with a client who is recovering from a severe trauma.

This theory, which I call "Bilateral Barrier Theory", is based on the recognition that *the six emotions of the grieving process serve to dissolve the natural barrier we put around trauma to protect ourselves from pain. This barrier dissolves over time so that our life force can enter the trauma to heal it when it is ready.* It all seems to make sense to me and I avidly go about creating charts and clinical aids that I use with clients in conjunction with Shape Therapy, which I have now relegated to the helpful position of one way to stimulate life force.

This new storm of creativity distracts me from my apprehension about leaving my material security. It also shows me, once again, that short of my wife and one best friend, there is no one to share my revelations with. The professional community is conservative and only allows itself to get excited over ideas which have been around for a while. I am alienated once again by their ignorance and, true to form, plunge into using my theory on clients without approval. The only feedback I am interested in is from my clients who seem to find my techniques useful. In this manner I am experiencing a tremendous amount of freedom and feel I am beginning to live the dream I projected a long time ago when I was inspired by Jung's autobiography. I don't care what my boss would say because I am planning to leave my job when the house sells and we move to the island. In a way I am giving over one responsibility (gainful employment) in favor of another (following my dreams and visions). I am spending all my spare time preparing for the move by building plywood boxes to house our art collection and selling off or distributing extra stuff we don't want to take with us.

Even though my wife does a fantastic job of fixing up the house, it seems to take forever to sell and we sometimes feel that we will never see our dreams come to fruition. Then, All of a sudden the house sells and we are faced with the chore of actually moving all our belongings to the coast.

In the old days I would have rented a truck, conscripted some friends and neighbors to help load, and moved it all by myself. Now we phone around and get a moving company to do it for us. We pack up the house and prepare for the day the movers will come. It feels very strange to watch the strong young men put little green tags (for insurance purposes) on every item in our household. I don't realize, until now, how grounding it is to keep in physical touch with our possessions during the process of moving. We have sent just about everything we own off in a truck to be stored in a warehouse until it can be delivered to a storage locker on Vancouver Island to await us while we search for a house on the little inner island we have now chosen to call home.

CHAPTER 27

BOXED IN

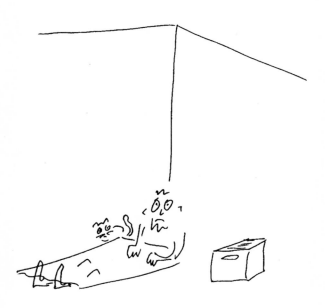

I still have to hang around the Okanagan and keep seeing clients for another couple of weeks until my responsibility to the job is complete. During this time we stay in a friend's basement as the new owners of our house are taking possession before we are able to leave town. This is very disturbing because I have come to rely heavily on a familiar home environment of my own creation to help me rebuild the image of myself as a householder. Floating in a strange house challenges my returning ability to deal with changing criteria. I am learning about the process of adapting to change by watching our big gray cat as he slowly expands his comfort level with seemingly disciplined explorations that lead him up through an unknown world and eventually out a window to the great outdoors.

After I have seen my last client, and we are packed and ready to leave, we set about preparing for the big drive to the coast. Even though we have shipped our household off to a storage locker there is still much to be packed in our smaller than compact sedan with the funky roof rack I installed over my wife's aesthetic protest. The car is overstuffed and the cat is given a knockout pill to keep him calm while we travel. He hates car trips and acts accordingly by yowling, thrashing about, vomiting, and pissing in his cage.

CHAPTER 28

WEIGHING ANCHOR

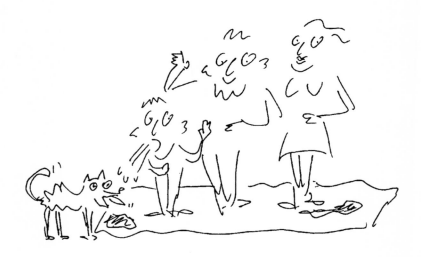

I am relieved when we are packed and ready to go. It is now, when I truly believe that the ordeal of getting ready is finally over, that my wife pleads with me to stop by a secondhand store to pick up a titty pink handmade wooden table she wants to take with us. She feels this table is a talisman of good luck and presses me to unload and reload my scientifically packed roof rack to make room for her treasure. Somehow I make the damn thing fit and we set off in a low riding Japanese tin can to meet our fate.

"He's dead!" my wife yells over the road noise bringing my attention to the comatose cat who probably, thanks to drug induced powers of astral projection, is already prowling the beaches of our island paradise to be. Ever the crisis junkie, I abruptly stop the car and leap into the back to examine my favorite feline. The cat looks stiff as a board with his tongue hanging out and his eyes rolled up in his head. An autonomic twitch assures me that he is still alive. I figure it's the knockout pill and we resume driving without further incident. But little do I know that, as we drive, my boy is building up a bilious brew in his stomach, which will later prove to be my daughter-in-law's undoing.

We are scheduled to spend the night at my second son's home in Victoria before we take off for the island. Plans are also made to rendezvous with old friends from California who will accompany us to a campground where we intend to camp until we find a house to rent or buy. I am dimly aware that our friends are bringing along a rambunctious new puppy to sleep with all the rest of us in my son's tiny living room and begin to dread the chaos.

We barrel into the well-kept apartment and find our friends already ensconced in the living room—puppy and all. After carefully setting up sleeping bags and laying out our night things we all get down to a California style back-to-the-land feast of Gargantuan proportions. This polyglot stuffing later inspires my boy's stomach to dump its contents all over wall-to-wall bags and blankets. My wife and I spring to the bathroom, raid some clean towels for mop-up, and fight the puppy for leftovers. This all proves too much for my daughter-in-law who barricades herself in the bathroom for the rest of our stay. I wonder if this bodes well for our new beginning and curl up in the middle of family, friends, and dogs. It is a testament to my returning health and the rightness of our choices that I don't experience any great anxiety over the physical discomforts that agitate the smoothness of our transition to the island. I am taking it all in stride with an ease and good humor that I only dreamed of since my accident.

CHAPTER 29

GEOGRAPHICAL CURE

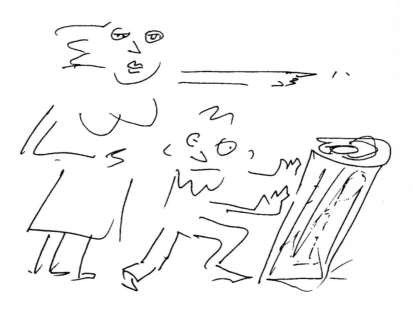

We roll into the campground to find a ten-pound package of pancake mix and a half gallon of fake maple syrup waiting on a heavy wooden picnic table—compliments of the Realtor who has anticipated our arrival by roping off a campsite right next to the ocean. It is glorious to be on the island with its beach and beautiful vistas and I begin to believe in the geographical cure.

Even though my excitement is dampened by an upset stomach, I manage to control mounting frustration over trying to figure out the telescoping poles and blithely help set up our new dome tents at the edge of the beach under some shade trees. It all looks too perfect to be real.

My wife is not satisfied with the efforts of our first encampment and has me busy switching sites. The tents move easily, as they are very light, but the chopping block up by the fire pit weighs a ton. I comment to the campers next door that I feel like a dung beetle rolling the damn thing back and forth as my wife fickles between the advantages of, what seems to me, two equally appointed campsites. She finally makes up her mind and we settle in to the obviously better nest. It doesn't occur to me to be a problem that we are now camped over 100 yards from the outhouses until I have discovered, too late in the evening, that my rumbling bowels have turned to water. My first night in paradise is spent crouching in ambulatory prayer between tent and outhouse. This nocturnal act of supplication helps me to pass our first night without soiling the bed— or my sweats. I have also managed to run both the men's and women's facilities clean out of toilet paper.

I am awakened by my wife's animated conversation with the campground attendant and his chuckling return that "someone must have had the runs real bad last night! both the shitters were stripped of paper!". "That was me!" I croak crawling out of the tent and offer him a hand that should be quarantined. Even in my depleted state I am very eager to make friends in our new community.

At the General Store the cashier asks me where I am from. It seems very natural for to me to answer "HERE!" She looks at me as if I am mad for she has never before seen me in her life and probably assumes that she knows everyone who makes their home on her small island. I have to admit the reflection from her eyes makes me feel a bit strange. This strangeness is not disturbing for it is *not* the strangeness from myself that I have been experiencing ever since my injury.

We develop a fine rhythm living on the beach waking up to spectacular sunrises and sandy beds. Creature comforts are hard to come by and
bird baths by the ocean, with water drawn and carried from the pitcher
pump well, make me feel cleaner than the civilized showers I left behind
in the Okanagan. I am finally shedding the persnickety skin that con-
tributed to keeping me a stranger from myself. There is some resistance
to this transformation and I am glad to be able to identify a positive shift
in my tolerance for dirt. I am not quite sure how to become an islander
and reach deep inside myself to hook onto the momentum of my wife's
vision. I will let the rest of my identity take care of itself.

CHAPTER 30

TRANSVESTMENT

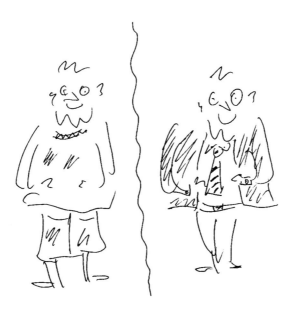

We meet locals at the beach and begin to establish friendships that lead to friendships that lead to a change of residence when we reach the limit of our stay in the provincial campground. This limit is set by the parks department and coincides with our ability to tolerate the scores of tourists who seem to be overrunning the campground. One of our new friends offers us a campsite in her orchard until a cabin on her property is vacant for our occupancy. We have been pursuing the purchase of a piece of property in the island's village core and, after having our offer accepted, are turned down for financing because I don't have a job. This is disappointing but we feel it may be for the best because we may need to live off our savings, which we have offered as a down payment until I do get work. Job interviews pop up as I answer adds in the local papers and begin to make connections on the big island (Vancouver Island). I get the interviews but nobody hires me. I still hold the dream that I can set up a private counseling practice on our small island.

In a couple of months we have to decide to find a larger rental because the cabin on our friend's property is too small to hold our household, which is still in a storage locker on Vancouver Island. I also want to find a place large enough to set up a home office.

I occasionally make pilgrimages to the locker at the request of my family to bring back vital pieces of our material puzzle necessary for our new life as it begins to unfold. The difficulty of this task is compounded by the fact that the movers packed the storage locker when they unloaded the truck and I have no idea where anything is. It just looks like the jumbled sea of an old familiar world flecked with little green tags.

My spiffy job interview clothes are carefully folded in a couple of suitcases I thoughtfully requested to be unloaded last. Sometimes I arrive at the locker looking like a beach bum and leave with the creased cuffs of a professional. The place is a dead row of closed garage doors and nobody witnesses the transvestment but me. I rejoice in this as a reflection of how flexible I have become. I am no longer solely relying on clues from my external world to tell me who I am. My inner sense of self is now strong enough to declare its person-hood, regardless of how I am dressed. After over ten years of being without a true personal identity, I am now ready to walk in the world conscious of my disguises.

When it comes time to move our stuff to the new rental I call up my son from Victoria, conscript some new friends, and rent a HUGE truck. All is pretty much like it was in the old days except that I don't do as much of the heavy physical work as I used to. I also manage to rake the virgin box of the brand new truck against a concrete filled pipe and miss more than a few shifts. I am definitely glad that I took out damage insurance on the truck. I am going to need it. We make our deposit on the island and move our stuff into the spacious new rental. I secretly yearn to own the place and feel myself phasing into the role of a real householder.

We set up a lower bedroom as a counseling office for me replete with its own telephone line and fancy new rug. After a couple of months of trying to drum up business I figure out that there just isn't enough of a population base on the island to build up a practice that can provide a living. Attempts to find jobs on the big island all fall through and we run out of money and are reduced to living on welfare. For some reason this does not depress me too much and I finally find myself with all the time in the world to follow my creative inclinations. I remember a time in the not-so-distant-past when I was also given this opportunity but was too depressed to do anything but lay my head down on the table.

Now I am able to create the momentum to voluntarily put my thoughts down on paper. I spend more and more time in my posh home office, with its new smelling rug, filling page after page with handwritten intellectual garbage. Some of this garbage seems profound enough to me to take the time and energy to put it into typewritten form. This presents a problem because I still don't think I can type or understand how to use a word processor. Every time I try to use a typewriter, I experience great frustration over the many mistakes I make. It all seems too much trouble and I would rather pay someone to do it for me.

CHAPTER 31

OLD DOG NEW TRICKS

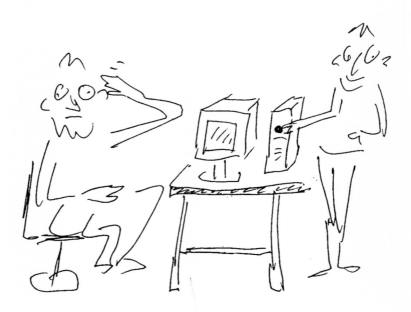

I hire a woman who has a word processor to type a seven-page paper for 7 dollars a page. I have to wait a couple of days for her to do the work and then drive across the island to pick up the manuscript. This arrangement is cumbersome and nets a finished product with several typos and paragraphs I would like to change. The woman is hard to reach by phone and I am feeling the need to get my paper in presentable shape—for what I don't know? It is raining outside and I feel stupid driving down dirt roads to find someone I can't reach by phone and spend another bunch of money to fix some typos on a paper I might want to revise as soon as I get home.

I would love to cut out the expensive and time consuming link between me and the printed word and am beginning to realize that there is only one way to do it. We have a computer upstairs that my son uses to play games and do homework. It has a printer and makes great copies. I am unemployed and have lots of time on my hands. I guess I'd better figure out how to use the damn thing.

One afternoon I ask my boy to show me how to turn it on. It is a step-by-step procedure that I scribble on a note pad and practice twenty or thirty times in a row. This is not easy for me. The computer only wants to be told how to operate in a stupid lock-step way. I feel extremely powerful when I finally get it to do what I want and relish the parade of numbers and letters that click before my eyes like a magic language and eventually end up as blank screen with a blinking cursor. Now I can practice typing and, more importantly, correct my mistakes. There is still much I don't understand but I have to start somewhere.

My boy, who has some facility with the machine, shows me the basic typing commands and I sit down one afternoon and begin to bang away at my seven-page paper. It is not easy and I discover major pitfalls in the path of my education. One is that I cannot rely on the boy to help me more than once when I get stuck. If I need more help after my first request, and his sometimes confusing explanation, he rages at me and dumps his resentment on me in the form of ferocious name calling and complete withdrawal of any aid at all. I feel terribly guilty about him having to help me and am forced to wait until he calms down. I have also discovered computer professionals in the community who have more patience with me and, with their help, manage to get around this very disturbing state of affairs.

It is also extremely hard not to give into the temptation to type only with my right hand but I plug away at it, with both hands, for hours and stagger off to bed at three o'clock in the morning, with twitching fingers and lines of words stamped on my mind. Something has broken loose in me and I feel a rare exhilaration as I begin on the path to mastery of a tool that will help change my life.

I take my newfound skills and create page after page of theoretical nonsense. There is no one to share it with except my wife who spurs me on. It is not really the content of what I write that matters but the fact that I am exercising my brain and developing more facility with the computer.

During this time I am invited to join an island writers' group because of my cartoon book. I don't consider it to be a particularly literary work but feel accepted as a fellow writer.

Some day I would love to write stories and maybe even a book. I have no idea how this could come about and continue to go to the group as a cartoonist.

One afternoon, while visiting some friends, I tell an ironic anecdote from my back-to-the-land days in California. My hostess is delighted and tells me I *must* do something with it. I am immediately inspired to reply that I will write it up for writers' group. In my mind I relish the task and feel confident to try my new computer skills out on such a project. Maybe this will help get my head out of my intellectual ass.

The story flows out of me and on to a fresh pad of lined paper. I write in pencil so that I can make corrections as I go along. Then I put it on the computer and make several layers of changes which bring it closer and closer to literary perfection. My wife is very taken with my work and tells me that I have quite a talent for writing. I can't wait to bring the story to writers' group and to create more. I madly jot down ideas for more stories and before I know it I am immersed in the creation of over twenty more. The writers' group encourages me and I find myself thriving on recreating incidents drawn from my rich and varied life *before* the accident. Each story has a drawing to go with it and I eventually put together a collection of illustrated short stories that I feel good enough about to send off to publishers. The publishers send me flattering rejection notices and I begin to develop an image of myself as a writer. This image is not at the exclusion of my profession as a counselor and I wonder when I might be blessed with the inspiration to put it all together.

CHAPTER 32

ONE MAGIC MOMENT

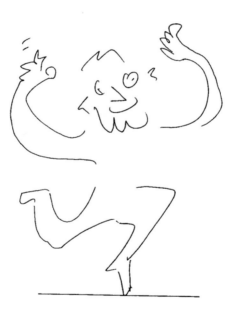

There finally comes a time when, after having written over thirty stories, I feel that I am running out of magical moments to recount. I am also tired of dwelling on events that happened to the *old* me. Where is the magic in my *new* life? I decide that it cannot be illuminated by isolated stories so I am forced to tell the whole tale.

I was born "*Dancing the edge*".

CHIP OFF THE OLD BLOCK

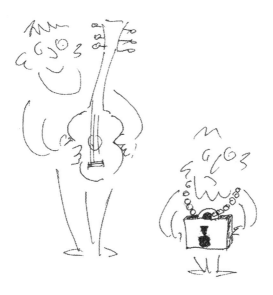

All these years, and all this healing.

We have left the inner island and moved to the beautiful city of Victoria on Vancouver Island. I am still counseling and writing and feel that I have reestablished a self-image that is meaningful, fulfilling, and fits with the activity of my life.

The "new" me does everything I could hope for, but play the guitar. Sure, I pick one up every once in a while and tumble out disjointed bits and remnants of my former competence. These spaced-out displays of ability flash me with nuggets of longing and unfulfilled potential. I still have weekly reoccurring dreams that I can play like I used to, and continue to grieve my losses throughout the day. The music is still within me but I have no way to get it out. And who better to be the instrument of its return than my youngest son who has decided, at the age of 22 that he wants to learn to play the guitar, and have me teach him everything I know? I guess this means I am going to have to go out and find him a guitar.

CHAPTER 34

STAIRYWAY TO HEAVEN

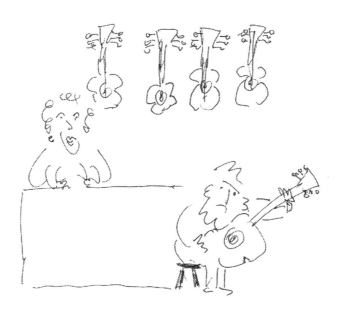

I have mixed feelings about shopping for a guitar. Part of me is excited with the prospect of finding and providing my boy with a sympathetic and inspirational instrument, and another part is terrified of exposing my musical ineptitude to the proprietors of guitar shops and/or other customers. Guitar shops are well-known for customers coming in and flexing their musical muscles on amateur versions of Lead Zeppelin's "Stairway to Heaven" and other standards. I don't think I can play any standards and feel musically breathless, flabby, and out of shape.

There is a little guitar shop in Fan Tan Alley where I occasionally go to pass time while my wife is shopping in Chinatown. I like the vibe of the place and come in to gently brush my thumb over the strings of the guitars hanging on the wall and listen to their voices—especially the older ones. I have been doing this for months, but never dare take one down to play. Now it looks like I will have to actually check a guitar for sound, action, intonation, and playability. This means taking it off the wall, sitting on a stool, and playing a few chords and melodic runs.

I ask the shopkeeper, a sparkly young woman with red hair, to take a couple down for me. Her presence behind the counter inspires my confidence as I sit on a stool curled over with my ear to the sound box softly strumming and fingering one of two guitars that I have chosen.

Though the guitar has a wonderful sound to my ear, playing it is a very unsettling experience and makes me feel sad, inadequate, and uncomfortable. I think that I should be thoroughly exercising this instrument in order to determine whether or not it is good enough for my boy. My discomfort turns to nervous chatter and I spill the whole story of my accident and loss of musicianship upon the proprietor's sympathetic ear. She doesn't say much, but witnesses the correctness of my choice by informing me that the guitar I have zeroed in on (a big, used, sunburst *Yamaha* dreadnought) is one that she often plays during slow times at the store, and is probably the best guitar that has come through the shop in a long time. I am thrilled with her response to my choice, as it tells me that I still have an ear for quality. I let her know that I might be back later to buy the *Yamaha* after I visit some other shops for comparison.

I feel off balance in the other shops I go to, and don't see or hear anything that compares favorably to my first choice. I am experiencing a distinct sweetness of anticipation and exhilaration as I contemplate returning to Fan Tan Alley to purchase the big *Yamaha* for my son. I also worry that it may have been picked up by someone else while I was out shopping around.

My wife accompanies me to Chinatown to make my purchase. I am relieved that the guitar is still in the store, and make the transaction of buying it with ease.

The *Yamaha* does not come with a case and I have to bring it to our car which is parked about a block away. I carry the instrument neck down, casually but carefully, for all to see and feel like a freewheeling Bob Dylan walking down the old city sidewalk with my beautiful wife on my arm.

CHAPTER 35

YOUNG DOG OLD TRICKS

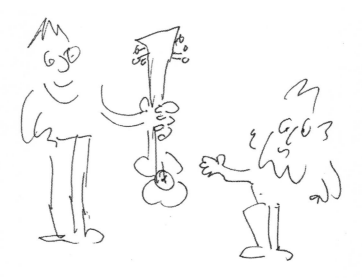

My son is delighted with his guitar and right away asks me to show him chords and runs. He is, by nature, an avid learner and picks up much of what I show him very quickly, then comes to me for more and more teaching. I tell him that I feel my demonstrations are fractured and describe them as a "bits and pieces of skillful playing that have been put in a box, shaken up, and sprinkled out at random". This perception is reinforced by the fact that we have only one guitar to play between us and the continuity of my demonstrations is hampered by handing the guitar back and forth.

Also there is no chance of playing together—which could be fun. Still, the boy makes great progress and asks me to show him something every time I see him.

My wife is heartened to see a musical relationship developing between me and my son and approaches me with the obvious next step in the process: It is time for me to buy myself a guitar so that I can more easily teach my eager student. This prospect puts me on the trail of an instrument that will match my sense of self-worth, image as a musician, and inspire me to play. I start poking around in the store where I bought my son's guitar, and take more than a few instruments off the wall in hope of finding something that meets my requirements.

Everything I choose to play, in my disjointed way, has potential, but nothing inspires me. I discover that I am looking for an instrument that is as experienced, beat up, mellow, and soulful, as I perceive myself to be—a tall order indeed.

I have heard of another store in town that sells a broader choice of new and used instruments including highly sought after and more expensive brands. I go there and do not feel like I belong in its rarified atmosphere. I am extremely shy about asking to play the beautiful and expensive guitars hanging on the wall. When I finally build the courage to ask about used instruments, the lowest price I am quoted is 700 dollars for a used guitar like the one I played before my accident. At this point I definitely do not feel that I am worth a 700 dollar guitar and decide to frequent some pawn shops to see if I stumble upon a less expensive guitar that meets my requirements.

The pawn shops have a desperate vibe and turn up a sparse choice of medium quality instruments that feel sad and seem overpriced. I keep going back to the store in Chinatown and almost buy an inexpensive guitar that plays easily and is well made, but doesn't have the rich sound that I long to hear. I am not sure what I expect to happen if and when I actually acquire a guitar, but I know I have to open myself up and surrender to the process of finding one.

CHAPTER 36

HAPPY TREES ON THE MOUNTAIN

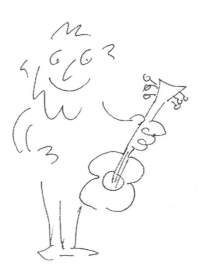

Slack times in my work schedule that used to be filled by sitting in coffee houses and window-shopping are spent browsing in every music shop I come across. One morning I find myself with some extra time to wander the streets while my car is being serviced at the mechanic's. I am surprised to see a small shop specializing in vintage guitars a short block or two from the garage. It is a fairly recent addition to the city and consequently unknown to me as a place to further my search. The shop is open and I enter as if there is nowhere else in the world for me to go.

The vibe is more relaxed than the store of expensive guitars and I sense the echoes of many songs emanating from some of the obviously well played and carefully restored instruments hanging on the wall. I am gently greeted by the proprietor and tell him that I am looking for a used guitar and would like to spend 300 dollars or less. He guides me to a row of older guitars that I recognize as good instruments of their time. I take down and strum a couple, then zero in on a big old dreadnought bodied *Yamaha* that sounds and feels pretty good, but is disappointingly flat in resonance and character. It is in good physical condition, evenly worn, and fully functional—but has mediocre tuning gears. I settle into a guitar stool and play very quietly to myself without much embarrassment as I am the only customer in the shop. The proprietor quietly watches me from the counter and then asks if I would be interested in trying out another guitar, within my price range, that is in the back room waiting to be cleaned up. This guitar is a 32 year old Japanese instrument named *Yamaki* that means "happy trees on the mountain". I am not aware of this brand as it was mostly imported, in the 1970's, into Canada during a time I was in The United States. When I strum this guitar it expresses the deep resonance that I have been seeking in an instrument. It seems in basically good shape, but has been abused by its previous owner(s) with sloppily applied black paint over its neck and several dents and small holes in its sides. The guitar still wears a coat of dirt and smells slightly sour, but manages to exude a subtle beauty that gleams through the years of careless use and abuse. I am moved by its sound and impressed by the high quality tuning gears that someone, sometime, saw fit to equip it with. I sit for a long time playing the big *Yamaha*, and then the *Yamaki*; one after the other, over and over.

The proprietor leaves me alone to make my own decision. I appreciate his sensitivity and respect for my process, then choose the *Yamaki* like jumping into the deep end of a pool and buy it feeling that I have just crossed a momentous bridge.

I also feel a great need to get rid of the terrible black paint that some-one applied so sloppily to the neck of my new guitar and ask the propri-etor if he has any suggestions on how to remove it. He tells me not to use any type of paint or varnish remover because it could corrupt a glue joint and encourage separation of the fingerboard from the neck. He instructs me to use fine sand paper and seal the neck with tung oil once I've removed all the paint. He also warns me that this type of sanding project is "not for the faint-hearted". I know from first hand experience that rehabilitation of the broken and neglected self is also not for the "faint-hearted.

MAKING IT MINE

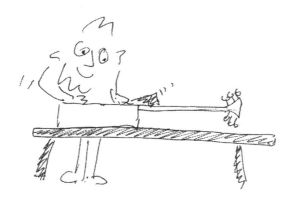

When I get the car back, I carefully place my new purchase in the trunk and drive home thinking that I must get to that black paint as soon as possible. It is like the work it will take to remove it stands between me and my rapprochement with music.

The black paint on the neck is impervious to my wife's "special formula" of turpentine and linseed oil and only begins to respond to being sanded, by slowly coming off as an ugly fine black powder a bit at a time. Each stroke brings me closer to having to play. Though the work is tedious, I am beginning to feel a sense of panic. It seems like the paint is embedded in the very pores of the wood! It takes great perseverance to reveal the natural finish of the neck under the paint and I contemplate attacking it with paint and varnish remover. I might have done so earlier in my recovery but now, after having gone back to school and written two full length books on rehabilitation, I perceive myself as a more patient and courageous man.

After several hours and many sheets of sandpaper I am starting to see more golden wood than smudgy black surface. The more I see, the faster it seems to go and somehow, miraculously, the neck is fully relieved of its black coating. Now I can apply tung oil in order to seal the raw wood. *I have the inner feeling that physically bringing this old guitar back to life is a metaphor for my own rehabilitation.* I am correct in this feeling, but the process has really just begun here in the basement.

My new guitar sounds great with a fresh set of strings and I begin to explore my ability to play with mixed reviews. I enjoy the sounds I am making but find it more difficult to make them than I expected. What did I expect? I know that I must start practicing every day and push through my disappointment like removing paint—a bit at a time.

THE SINGER NOT THE SONG

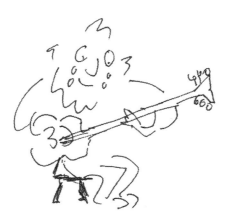

I close myself in my room (office/studio) and struggle to play day after day. It actually sounds like I am getting marginally better after about a week but I continue to ravage the fingers on my left hand which have completely lost the player's calluses that I took for granted twenty years ago. The pain, which might be normal for beginners, seems amplified by injury related confusion of the sensory nerves in my hand and plagues me with a variety of distracting tinglings and pulsations for hours after I stop playing. I am committed to the project and begin to think that making my guitar play easier might be a way out of my suffering. I take the guitar to a luthier who is reputed to be the best in town and happens to be at the store of expensive guitars. He carefully looks over the instrument and tells me that it will need about 400 dollars of work to put it in order. He also recommends against the work saying that, in his opinion, the guitar is not worth the price of repairs. It is like *he is telling me that I am not worth fixing*. I do not want this man, no matter how good his reputation, to work on my guitar if he does not appreciate the qualities that have drawn me to it. I am deeply offended and ask him to send me to another member of his profession. He vouches for an associate who happens to have a workshop in my home neighborhood.

The second luthier looks over the old *Yamaki* and explains why he thinks his colleague devalued my guitar ("too busy with more expensive guitars"). He says he believes my guitar is well worth the cost of repairs. I do not leave the guitar with him for repairs, but say that I will let him know when I am ready to have them done.

My wife is not impressed with my plan to spend more money on my new instrument to make it play more easily. She tells me that she will only support such expenditure if I practice with the instrument in its present condition until I find my technique improving as a result of my own efforts. Then, and only then, will she be comfortable spending more on my guitar. I am mildly disappointed but appreciate her wisdom in helping me make the distinction that it is *I* who need the work and not the instrument. Her response has also encouraged me to value my efforts and reward them with repairs when we feel I have earned them.

I daily pit myself against the brutal steel strings for the next four months and eventually find myself playing better and better with less pain and effort. I also feel very emotional and sometimes cry as I strum familiar chords and relive old songs and melodies. I know that I do not play with my pre-injury confidence and ease but deeply enjoy my time making music. I don't have to be great for anyone anymore—just enjoy the sweet sounds. Now I can approach my wife about bringing my guitar up to my ability to play.—a much different request from fixing up my guitar to make me play better. She has been listening to me through the door of my office and agrees that it is time to have the instrument repaired.

CHPATER 39

THE LONG WAIT

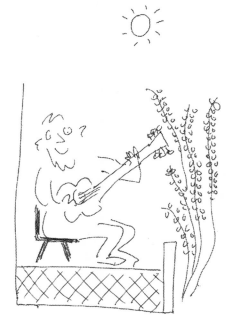

The second luthier takes my guitar giving me an estimate of two and one half weeks to make the repairs we have agreed upon. It really takes twice as long as estimated and I almost go crazy with anticipation of playing my fixed-up guitar. I borrow a guitar from my oldest son who lives in town so that I can keep up my daily practice. The tone of my borrowed instrument is not as enchanting as that of "happy birds on the mountain" but I overcome this lack and keep playing every day mixing my impatience with the sweet expectation of having the *Yamaki* returned to me in better condition.

I finally get the call that my guitar is ready and race to the luthier's to pick it up. He shows me his work and tells me that it was one of his most gratifying repairs because the old guitar responded well, with improved clarity and tone, after getting a new saddle and nut, having the frets dressed, some loose braces re-glued, and the action properly set up. I am delighted and take my guitar home to discover that my left hand is somewhat of a stranger to the fretboard after having adjusted its proprioception to the narrower neck of my son's guitar. This alerts me to the nature of my remaining disability and helps me adjust my playing style to allow for the fact that, thanks to my injury, the fingers of my left hand have a very limited ability to form a memory of where they are in space. I have learned, from reading Oliver Sacks, that proprioception is dependent on the visual sense as well as neurological activity, and that I can compensate for my compromised neuro-pathways by looking at my fingers. Now I look at my fingers as I play. The more I play, the less I have to look, but it's definitely not pre-injury automatic anymore.

I still play shut up in my office or *very* quietly to myself on the back porch when the weather allows. I wonder what the neighbors think, if they hear me. I am shy and don't quite feel ready to play in front of or with others in spite of the fact that I am beginning to sound pretty good to my own ear.

Why did it take *twenty years* to be able to accept this change in ability? I am no longer bummed out by the indisputable fact that I do not play with as much confidence and dexterity as I did before my brain injury. This is probably because I have developed a self-image that is not centered on my abilities as a musician. I resisted this change of self-image as long as I felt the need to grieve the loss of those abilities. It took *twenty years of grieving* to accept myself as I am. Now I see myself as a creative being who is a counselor, writer, cartoonist and musician. I love sharing all these facets of myself and am beginning to feel that I want to play with others.

CHAPTER 40

OUT OF THE CLOSET

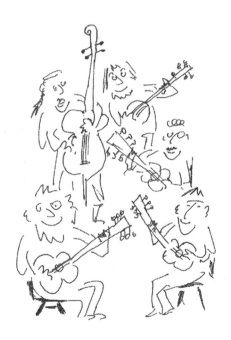

One of my neighbors, who seems like a sympathetic person, and has even read the first edition of this book, casually mentions that he plays the banjo. I think that it might be fun to see if I can keep up with accompanying him on simple folk and country tunes that don't have too many chord changes. He is agreeable and we set up a date to play together in his converted garage.

Playing with the banjo proves to be as delightful as I predicted and we start and maintain weekly get-togethers that have expanded beyond simple banjo tunes to include old folk songs that he and I know from our past. We are even building a warm and respectful friendship around our newfound musical relationship. This relationship gives me confidence and I contemplate attending a weekly bluegrass "jam" I have heard about that is put on by a local bluegrass association. The association's website recommends coming and listening before participating.

I summon courage and drive out to a little wooden church hall that houses the association's activities. I feel more confident seeing other folks walk towards the building carrying guitar, mandolin, and violin and banjo cases. A middle aged woman falls in beside me on the pilgrimage from car to church and asks me how long I have been playing. I respond, "About 55 years, with a long time out of 20 years", and do not feel the need to tell her about my car accident. She informs me that the jams are not difficult and nobody really minds if you stumble along, as long as you don't play too loudly. This makes sense and I overcome some anxiety and begin to look forward to the experience.

The hall is filled with 20 or more musicians sporting a number of guitars, mandolins, banjos, violins, dobros, and two stand-up basses.

Chairs are set up in a circle and everyone takes their instruments out of their cases and finds a seat. Then they begin to warm up by playing to themselves a bit before someone declares that he or she wants to play a particular song and everyone joins in. Some of the folks play really well, but there are no obvious virtuosos here and no one strives to stand out above the crowd. The music is straightforward and sounds like it is within my ability to chord along. After about fifteen minutes of listening I feel a curious mixture of confidence mixed with the desire to play, and then walk out to the car to get my guitar.

I have to work very hard for the next two hours to keep up with the chord changes that, though simple, seem like they are coming at me rapid-fire. Nobody glowers at me while I am playing and I am not asked to leave the building, so I guess I am doing alright. It seems a miracle that I am not put off by my limited ability to play these simple tunes that used to be so easy, and am satisfied just making music with others. I truly enjoy playing the guitar for the sake of playing even though the fingers of my left hand hurt like hell.

When I get home I am tired like after a strenuous physical workout. I know that playing tonight must have been good therapy for my brain because I go to bed, with smoking ears, running chord changes over and over in my mind before I fall asleep.

I continue to go to the Tuesday night jams and have become a regular attendant. Some nights are better than others and it takes a while for me to identify and become friendly with other regulars whom I particularly enjoy playing with.

I am now playing music two nights a week. Once with my neighbor across the street and again at the bluegrass jam. I also practice at least a half hour each day to increase my skills and keep my fingers tough. I need to keep in shape for making music with my son who brings his big *Yamaha* along when he comes to visit. We play together for hours. It is great fun.

Another new friend has invited me to several musical gatherings and I helped a neighbor restore a neglected guitar so it seems that I am beginning to have a lot on my musical plate. I have also found a discarded high-quality stereo receiver on the street which I have refurbished and combined with good hand-me-down speakers and a used turntable. Now I am able to surround myself with music while I work on my other endeavors.

My wife has put her foot down and only lets me out of the house to play music twice a week so she does no become a musician's widow like she was for 20 years in the old days. This is good for me so I can divide my energy more equally between all of my creative interests.

The nature of my improvement on the guitar is interesting in its unfolding. I seem to be getting better at knowing when to change chords and am even beginning to be able to anticipate what chord to change to. My rhythm is becoming more trustworthy and I can shift my rhythmic emphasis without getting lost, however the dexterity and proprioception of my left hand still seems to be lagging behind. I have faith that it will improve with more practice and push myself through funky sounding efforts that result from painful fingertips and uneven pressure on the fret board.

I am even able to play a couple of songs from start to finish, but do not feel confident to perform them for anyone other than some close friends and my banjo buddy across the street. My wife says my singing sounds terrible and is not improving along with my ability to play the guitar. I suppose that I will have to either sing only for myself and get really good on the guitar without singing—or start the journey back to finding my singing voice. Maybe, some day, I'll be able to artfully use my vocal chords again. It remains to be heard.

CHAPTER 41

HOOTENANNY

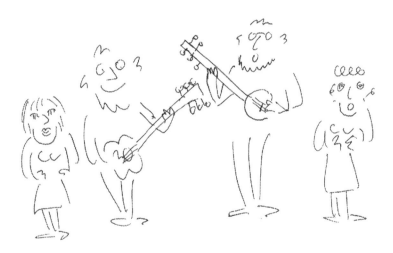

My wife and the wife of my musical compatriot across the street have decided to get us all together for dinner and an after dinner concert featuring me on guitar and my friend on banjo. We hope to have about five songs ready for performance and I suffer great waves of performance anxiety. My buddy tries to soothe my nerves by describing the women as the "toughest and most supportive" audience we could ever hope to have. This description both frightens and heartens me at one and the same time. We spend our last rehearsal before the "show" honing our best five songs and actually begin to feel like we have something to offer the women.

The evening of the event arrives like the ring of doom and I go across the street carrying my guitar like a death-row convict carrying the hanging rope. Dinner is enjoyable and I exert self-control not to gorge myself on the good food so I am not too full to play comfortably after we eat.

Our first couples of songs go surprisingly well and the audience seems delighted with the music in spite of some gross mistakes on both our parts. We complete our repertoire and are easily coaxed to play many requests which we warm to more easily than we expected. I am delighted to hear my wife singing along and thrilled to hear her say out loud that she feels that it is "like it used to be in the old days". But, these are the "new days" and she is even tolerating me croaking along with my buddy who takes most of the lead vocals. This evening's show goes down in the neighborhood hall of fame and we plan to get together for more musical get-togethers and master another five songs for next time.

It has been almost exactly a year since I started playing again. I have also just ceased having reoccurring weekly dreams that I could play the guitar with pre-injury facility—only to be disappointed, upon waking, that my abilities were still compromised. These dreams were so realistic and vivid that I wondered if my ability to play wasn't locked inside me with no way to get out.

It is now clear that the process of my neurological healing combined with grief through, denial, sadness and anger over not being able to play like I used to took 20 years to heal me to the point where I am again able to explore and enjoy the music that is so dear to me.

I am not how I used to be before my injury but have recovered something I thought was lost forever—and I thought you'd like to know that it can come full circle.

PS. We have added a violin player to our neighborhood duo and expanded our repertoire to include some jigs and reels.

Part II

Inside Brain Injury

Introduction To Part II

You have just read a firsthand account of my experience with brain injury. It was written to stand alone as a memoir that tells a very personal and unique story. It is my hope that this story will help others understand and relate to the experience of losing and regaining self-image.

Through contact with survivors of brain injury as a helping professional, I have become more aware that much of my story is unique to my own personal experience. I have also observed that the psychological process of coming to terms with the loss of my self-image, and consequent quest to establish a new one, is fundamental to the nature of my injury and virtually all those I have worked with.

Some of what I am writing about is drawn from my own experience, and some from clinical experience with numerous clients who have shown endless variation in manifesting symptoms and behaviors associated with their injuries.

Part II is written in a manner that I hope makes understanding how it feels and what it means to be brain injured more accessible for use in the recovery process. It is written directly to the survivor, but addressed to family, caregivers, and professionals who may wish help the survivor understand what has happened to them.

First Knowledge of Trauma

To the Caregivers

It is my hope that this section of the book will help you, the caregivers, understand how to cope with a brain injury as if you had suffered one. It is not necessarily meant to be read, by all survivors (especially in the early stages of their recovery). Some survivors will be in too great a state of denial and some will be too confused or plagued by cognitive disabilities to be able to comprehend sequentially written material. Some may have lost their use of language altogether and may need to be approached, with this text much later in their recovery, after they have regained some facility with language and the ability to comprehend sequential material. If they are able, curious, and willing, by all means offer this chapter right away. Alternately, you may choose to save this chapter for later, or read only the preceding memoir, like a story, out loud, to help your survivor know that he or she is not completely alone in their experience. Subsequent chapters may be read to and by survivors to help them through later stages of their recovery.

Waking Up

When you first come to consciousness after an injury to your brain, providing you have experienced some level of unconsciousness, you may feel disoriented and not know how, or when, you got to where you perceive yourself to be. This would ordinarily feel very uncomfortable, but after an injury to your brain, you are not in an ordinary state of mind. The uncomfortable part of disorientation is probably masked by your feelings of childlike surrender to your situation.

Take it Easy

In this state of mind, there is not much else to do but just go with the flow. Relax, don't concern yourself with how you got to where you are, and don't push yourself to make up the time you feel you have lost. These missing markers in your time-space continuum may become available to you again when your brain has healed enough to be able to reassemble the broken pieces of your experience in an understandable manner. This often takes longer than you think.

The Myth of Willpower

Neurological healing is very slow and has a pace and mind of its own. It also does not respond well to therapies that stress the exertion of your will to heal. You may, in fact, feel violated by someone pressuring you to help yourself through exerting your will power before you are able.

Before you blow up at them, explain that the process of recovery from brain injury is much different than the process of recovery from physical injury, and that *figuring out how your will is connected to you* is at the core of your rehabilitation. Then tell them that you might consider employing willpower to help you heal once you have reconnected it to your sense of self.

Remembering What Happened

You may need the help of family, friends, or professionals to reclaim some memory of your trauma—or you may never retrieve the lost parts of your memory. Either way it is nothing to concern yourself with in the immediate days, weeks, or months following injury to your brain. Pushing to know exactly what happened to you, when you are not ready or able to understand it, can only cause you unnecessary grief. There is nothing you can do about it—and it really doesn't matter! Your job is to be as comfortable as you can in the present.

Relating to Caregivers

In this world, you do not live in a vacuum and are most likely surrounded by loved ones and caregivers who are motivated by love and professional dedication to want to help you recover from your injuries. You did not ask for their presence in your life and may find them strange, troublesome, or hard to relate to. This is because you don't know where to place them in your world. Don't expect to love all your caretakers. Many of them will not know how to relate to you. Others may fulfill deep emotional needs and offer you the right help at the right time. You can be expected to be confused, weepy, or grumpy, and may have to wait for your caregivers to learn how to relate to you while you rebuild your world.

Caregivers may experience frustration with your seemingly unrealistic interpretation of what happened to you, and it is advisable for them *not* to pressure you to remember the circumstances of your injury—especially if you show confusion and distress over trying to remember. Caregivers may, and should, offer a calm, grounded, and factual account of the circumstances surrounding an injury *only* if you trust and feel good about them. What you hear may upset you and inspire you to ask more questions, so your caregivers have to be prepared to handle your potentially extreme emotional responses to information that triggers uncomfortable parts of your memory.

Don't Shoot the Messenger

Not every emotional response makes sense in brain injury survivors, and it is good to remember that the emotion you express over hearing the truth about your injuries has not been caused by the caregiver who is trying to orient you to your situation. Caregivers are only messengers of facts that you may perceive as hurtful and confusing. In this role they are in perfect target position for a classic "shoot the messenger" set-up and are not your enemies, nor deserving of your rage and disappointment. Your caregivers must keep this in mind and not feel personally attacked, even though the negative emotion displayed seems like it is directed precisely at them.

Relating to Family

You may not know or recognize members of your family as people you are close to. *This is much harder for them than it is for you.* Your inability to identify them, as loved ones, is extremely distressful for them because they love you and are most likely very attached to you. They want to help you and expect you to be able to relate to them in order to do so. You are not rejecting them by not remembering them, but simply cannot place them in your world because it has been shattered by your injury. You may have lost your sense of who you are, and along with it, some, if not many, of your most important connections to the world—including your family.

Family and Strangers

You, on the other hand, may feel a familial connection with strangers, including professional caregivers whom you have never met before. This is because you have lost the ability to keep your world in order and have taken to filling lost connections, or gaps in your memory, with people and places that remind you of the missing parts. Your family may find it distressing, especially if you cannot recognize them, and professionals may be confused, but you will eventually get it sorted out as your brain heals and possibly laugh about it later when you have figured out "who's on first".

Facing your Situation

The reality of the disabling nature of your injuries may be so over-whelming that your first response is to deny that they ever happened to you. You have awakened to a body and mind that don't work like they're supposed to, and more importantly you feel so alienated from the world that it is easy to believe that your broken body does not belong to you any more! This feeling will decrease as your nerves heal, but will always remain with you as you get used to hauling around parts of your body that have a mind of their own.

Losing Touch with Your Body

Not belonging to your body is a convenient way to disassociate your-self from your situation, and a sure symptom of injury to your nerves. There is nothing you can do about it right away and, like losing your place in time and space, you have to wait for a certain degree of healing to occur before you can expect to regain any connection with your lost parts.

Early Denial of Injury

You may have the feeling that nothing bad has happened to you and that you still retain all your powers. This feeling is so deeply seated that it flies in the face of your serious disablement. This is because *you are used to experiencing yourself as a whole person and don't quite feel like one.* You have lost your image of yourself as a complete functioning per-son and will deny, at all costs, that you have really lost any part of your functioning.

To overcome this denial, and begin to really rehabilitate, you must learn to perceive yourself as whole, even though your injured brain has destroyed your ability to do so. This is possible through a process of reminiscence that *prepares* you to grieve your old life.

Reminiscing

Immerse yourself in old pictures, tapes, or photo albums, and re-familiarize yourself with successfully completed projects and triumphs. You may find yourself shedding a lot of tears and remembering yourself as the greatest_____there ever was. This may or may not be true, but it is the closest, at this time, that you can get to experiencing yourself. It is the only intact self-image your brain has left and you probably won't be able to begin to come to terms with losing it until you re-experience it on some level.

Losing Memory of Yourself

Loss of memory is often associated with brain injury and can greatly contribute to the feelings of confusion and disassociation that you may feel upon discovering yourself in a changed condition. Though it can also serve to insulate you from knowledge of the seriousness of your condition, it can be, in itself, a great cause for dread and dismay.

Familiar Music

You may find that complex music, videos and reading material brought to you by family or caregivers, do not comfort you or provide a welcome distraction because they don't make sense like they used to. This can be very unsettling if you desperately want and need entertainment to distract you from your injuries and surroundings (hospital or recovery center). What you get from these well-intended distractions is the opposite of comfort: confusion and the frightening feeling that you have lost an important connection with your world.

If you feel yourself becoming disconnected from your world because you cannot remember one moment from the next, a good thing to do is immerse yourself in familiar, predictable, repetitive music (of your choice), through headphones, which provides you with a stable predictable time flow that does not tax your memory. As you heal, and come out of the first shock of consciousness after injury, you may find that your memory will gradually return and you will be able to develop strategies to compensate for loses you may be left with. Further discussion of problems with memory can be found later.

CHAPTER 2

Trying To Find Yourself

Common wisdom, in the field of neurology, is that you will probably get as back to normal as you are going to get in ten years. I like to extend this period to fifteen, and look at it in five-year increments with healing progress being most dramatic in the first year, and getting more and more subtle as time goes on. You can have a life while you are working towards your point of full recovery, though you may find yourself distracted by comparisons to how you used to be. This is okay because it is part of your healing process. I believe that you will continue to heal well beyond what is called the point of full recovery (15 years). It may be unsettling to realize that you will never be your old self again but you will eventually regain, as a new person, the sense of wholeness you feel you have lost.

Going Home

When you are in a hospital or recovery center you probably want nothing more than to return home and resume your life. Going home from the hospital has become a major focus and you will agitate for it until you have received your wish. Going home is the best possible thing for you, when you are physically able and have been provided with appropriate support systems in your home and community.

Support Systems at Home

Support systems include setting up and maintaining relationships with home support workers and medical, physical, occupational, and counseling professionals. Successful reentry to your home may also include the refitting of your house with any improvements and aids you need to help you gain your best level of physical independence.

The setting up of this home/community support system is not your responsibility and should be manifested, in consultation with the professionals in charge of your transfer to home and community. You can help them by being as clear and realistic as you can about what you want and need to be able to do in your home to make you feel real.

Controlling Your Environment

In a hospital, or recovery center environment, you may feel that you have no control over your environment because it does not reflect anything that you can relate to as part of your self-image. Visitors, including family, may seem weird and distant to you and may try to relate to you as you *were*. Be yourself. It is not your responsibility to change for them. They are visitors, who wish you well and need to learn to adapt to your new way of being.

Different Than You Used To Be

You will deny to yourself that you are different from what you used to be and insist, in spite of reflections of your changed condition, that given the opportunity to do_____again, you would become as you were—"No problem!" This is a normal psychological response to a brain injury at this stage because your self-image is stuck at a pre-injury state and yearns for an environment that can give you the comfort and feedback of knowing who, and where you are in the world.

You believe, in the strongest way, that you will feel out of sorts until you return home—and maybe even magically return to yourself when you are in familiar surroundings. As much as you think you will bounce back to yourself, when you come in the front door, *you will not*. I do not say this to sound cruel, or hopeless, but it is my experience, both as a survivor and professional caregiver, that *the shock of trying to impose the totality of your old life on a new and incomplete self-image can be a very unsettling experience.*

Coming Home

Now that you have gotten your wish, and are back in your familiar home environment, you may be very distressed to discover that you feel like you don't belong there. How can this be? You spent a lifetime building the relationships with your world that made you *feel* real! It will take you some time to reconnect your feelings to a new way of being.

Managing Your Affairs

If you feel like you don't fit in your world anymore, you probably are not able to manage your affairs. This makes you dependent on caregivers for your survival, and takes a great toll on your level of self-confidence, which is rapidly eroding as you despair of ever being able to support yourself again.

Your despair, though very real and understandable, is not helpful for your condition. *Your job is to heal and its returns are infinitely greater and more appropriate for your condition than those of the illusion of self-sufficiency you cling to in search of your old self.* You really have no idea what your life will bring you when you recover and emerge as a new person.

You will never feel the same again and are beginning to realize that you have embarked on a particular journey of self-discovery for which you have had no preparation. The last time you created a self-image you did it as a child. Now you are forced to create one in the shadow of the person you were.

CHAPTER 3

Grief And Brain Injury

The Grieving process is the way we heal from our experience of loss. It provides us with a way to emotionally process change in our lives and gradually come to terms with how it affects us. Change is only perceived as negative if it takes away something that we have formed an attachment to. Probably the most difficult thing to separate ourselves from is our image of ourselves. We would never choose to make this separation, even if we hated ourselves, because we have been trained (and tricked) by our culture to completely identify with how we think the world perceives us.

You have suffered a brain injury and   t your pre-injury image of yourself. Losing your self-im   the most difficult thing your can lose in this world. Righ   ising your life. The only way to heal from such a loss is th   g process.

This means you must feel shock (n   s, anger, fear, denial and guilt so that you can process you   tions are appropriate to grieving in most circumstances bu   inings and conditions if you have had a brain injury, whi   ter an examination of the function of each grieving emoti...   iecessarily come in any order with one emotion following another but show up to help you process your loss as you need them. You may need a counselor or therapist to help you through the grieving cycle without harming important relationships, or yourself.

Shock

Shock, or numbness, is most likely to turn up first when you have lost something because there usually is a period of delay between the sharpness of a loss and the pain you will feel about it. You need to allow yourself time, without intense pain, for your emotions to adjust for your loss. Numbness can also come later to help you shut down and rest between stronger emotions that may follow.

It is good not to let yourself become stuck in a state of numbness because, even though you are feeling no pain, you are keeping yourself from recovering by holding off the other emotions that you *must* go through to heal.

Shock and Brain Injury

The shock to the system that a brain injury produces may be confused with the grieving emotion of numbness. You will be stunned by the separation from yourself that you experience upon suffering a brain injury. It is *not* grief that you are feeling but a combination of the physical and psychological sledgehammer that has assaulted you on many levels. This assault is so profound, that you may not be able to feel anything about it other than the shock of not feeling like yourself at all.

Remedy for Shock

The best remedy for dealing with the type of shock that comes from a brain injury, is to *know that your natural healing processes have immediately kicked into gear to heal you, and are already busy with the work of bringing you back to health.* If you don't have someone you trust to tell you this, you may not believe it, but it may be the most important bit of information you will ever hear and lead you, from numbness, to a state of real confidence in your ability to heal.

Sadness

Sadness is an emotion that you have probably experienced in your life, and provides a rich opportunity to re-live how you felt before, during, and after you sustained a loss. It is appropriate to feel sad about losing _____, but dangerous to repress your feelings because they can fester inside you and become depression, which is a much more serious and disabling condition.

Sadness and Brain Injury

If you have had a brain injury, your expression of the vulnerability you feel at having been stripped of your self-image may be mistaken for sadness. You may cry and seem morose when you are only acting as you would if you were a lost child trying to comprehend "What has happened to me?"

When you suffer a brain injury, you probably have a lot to feel sad about because you may have lost, what you perceive to be, *your whole life*, including control, mobility, talents, abilities, livelihood, and lifestyle. These are HUGE losses and, because you have undergone more than one at a time, you will most likely feel very devastated and desperate. Sadness is an obvious response and it is good to *remember not to grieve all your losses at once*. If you do, you will be overwhelmed and risk the chance of falling into a depression.

Remedy for Sadness

Take your losses one at a time, and say to yourself: "*I am sad about losing my_____*" *(one loss only)*. This will keep you from falling into the trap of saying, "I am sad", or worse yet, "I am sadness!" It is appropriate to feel sad *about* losing something—but saying that you are sadness itself is to court a severe and disabling depression.

Anger

Anger is usually looked at as a separate emotion and overlooked as a healthy expression of grief. This is because it always has a negative effect on others and should not be allowed to destroy relationships. As an emotion of grief, anger provides much the same means for re-living and processing loss as sadness, denial, fear, and guilt.

Anger and Brain Injury

With a brain injury, frustration is often confused for anger and relationships unnecessarily suffer because people close to you think that you are raging at them when they are merely in the path of your frustration. You have much to be frustrated about because, due to your injury, your body and mind are not behaving like you want them to—sometimes even your feelings are out of control. What might have previously registered as displeasure with a frustrating task, or situation, has now become a battleground for your fight to comprehend and control your world. People around you are not soldiers in the war you are having to gain control of yourself and consequently are not there to be fired upon.

You will find that anger control strategies, like counting to ten, or leaving the room before you explode, might be useful but do not always work well for anger born of frustration. If you wish to get a better handle on your anger, you can explore community or professionally provided resources such as anger management courses or workshops. *The intensity of your outbursts will diminish as you become more comfortable with your limitations and incorporate them into your new self-image.* Your screams will recede to muttered curses. Unfortunately, no matter how you express your frustration, you are bound to affect people around you negatively.

Remedy for Anger

It is recommended, as with sadness, to take your losses one at a time. Say to yourself: "*I am angry about losing* _____ ". This will keep you from falling into the trap of saying "I am angry" or worse yet, "I am anger!" Even though it is not well accepted in our culture, to show anger, it is appropriate to feel angry *about* losing something—but saying that you are anger itself is to court rage and risk seriously harming others or yourself.

Redirecting Anger

It is very important that you make it clear to anyone you may have hurt with your response to frustration, that *you are not angry at them, but only releasing tension over something that has nothing to do with them.* Apologies can go a long way towards healing the hurt you may have caused.

Fear

Fear is sometimes called the source of all our negative emotions. It can be devastating and is capable of crippling our lives and freezing our progress. As an emotion of grief it provides the function, if held within bounds, to re-live your losses in a vivid and meaningful manner.

Fear has a way of preying on a single aspect of a loss by taking over your life with a specific dread. It can paralyze your progress but is really, as an emotion of grief, trying to lift your burden of loss through helping you to know yourself better. You can work with fear to help you grieve by examining it closely in order to see what it is trying to teach you. It will often give you clues about how it is making you re-live your loss.

Pay attention to what exactly it is that is making you afraid. The connection to your loss may be obscure, and you may need aid from a friend, counselor, or therapist to help you figure it out. Put on the attitude of a detective and ask yourself "Where is the connection between my fear and my loss?" How is it helping me re-live my relationship to it?" You will be amazed how this ominous emotion can help you work through your grief. Once you have solved the mystery of what your fear is telling you about yourself, you will be better prepared to deal with it when it crops up again to teach you more.

Fear and Brain Injury

Fear may not seem as much of a problem after a brain injury as it did before, because there is not much more that can happen to you after losing yourself—a situation similar to losing your life. In fact, *very much the same as losing your life—without experiencing physical death*. Some injuries produce comas, and others may be the result of loss of oxygen to the brain, which is a type of physical death. You probably don't remember your coma if you had one, and therefore still don't know what it was like to be "dead"—so fear of death may still remain an issue for you. It is probably best left to deal with after you have regained more self-image and can approach it with a more solid knowledge of yourself.

The terror you may feel in losing your time and place in the world, due to severe injury to your memory, is not fear but terror which is generated by having lost all security in this life. This injury specific response may be completely out of your control and is best dealt with by allowing trusted friends, members of your family, and professionals to re-anchor you in this world through therapy designed to restore your memory.

There is also the terror that comes from Post Traumatic Stress which is the result of unresolved response to trauma. It is derived from suppression of memory, and will be discussed later as a specific event.

Remedy for Fear

One way of finding out what part of your loss your fear is connected to is to ask yourself: "*I am afraid of* _____—*just like* _____". How you fill in the "just like" part of the equation will give you a more specific indication of what you are grieving by being afraid. You might say, for example, "I am afraid of having another stroke, *just like* the one I got in my accident!" This gives you the opportunity to process your accident, with its attendant losses, one more time without being overcome by fear itself.

Denial

Denial functions much like the other emotions of grief as a means to help you process loss by re-living it through denying that it ever happened to you. It may seem paradoxical that by trying to say that your loss never happened, you are creating a space to re-live it in your mind, but it is so. Every time you tell yourself "this never happened", you are providing yourself with the opportunity to contemplate the "this" that never happened.

Denial is as tricky as it is helpful because, like numbness, it can lure you into a false sense of well being and fool you into not being realistic about your condition. This can create great physical or emotional problems, as you attempt to go about acting like a completely functional person without the ability to do so. You can imagine what kind of trouble you could get yourself into if you tried to fly with your wings before they grew feathers.

Denial and Brain Injury

Denial with a brain injury is not the denial of grief, but a subject unto itself. It is a way for you to feel complete after you have lost your self-image. *When you deny that you have lost your powers, and say to yourself that you are "like you used to be", you are jumping back to the only sense of wholeness that you have: your image of yourself before your injury.*

It may frustrate your family and caregivers to hear you go on and on about how you "*used to be the greatest* _____", and if you "*could only do or have* _____*again*", then you "would be alright". It is not a bad idea to take all the time you need to talk about the past. Feeling powerful in remembrance is good for you because it helps solidify whatever image of yourself you retain as a foundation for creation of the new one.

Just remember that what you feel you can do, and what you actually can do are two different things. You may get furious when caregivers deny you access to activities that could endanger lives (even yours) but don't stop asking them to let you do new things. You may be surprised at how you can grow by pushing your boundaries if you give thought to those around you. Remember you will suffer bitter disappointment when you come up against not being able to perform tasks that used to be easy, or even natural for you.

Take your defeats as gracefully as you can, even after you have cried or screamed about them, and remember that you will master wonderful new talents, as your new self, that you never dreamed of before your injury. You may also regain old abilities that you think you have lost— but not all of them.

Remedy for Denial

The best way to deal with a trickster, is to outsmart it by not buying into its trick. Therefore you must keep in mind, at all times, that *every time you are denying your loss you are making it exist so that you can grieve it.* Denial will then cease to lull you into a false sense of power, and begin to realistically inform you about your condition.

Guilt

Guilt is another emotion of grief that functions by helping you re-live your loss through contemplating your relationship to it. The emotion of guilt, in grieving, is not the same as feeling guilty or being guilt stricken. Again, like fear, it has a very specific range of usefulness to grief. It challenges you to take responsibility for your actions, even though it is too late, and forces you to suffer through the choices that were available to you at the time of your loss.

Guilt and Brain Injury

Guilt is not a grieving emotion that you may feel after suffering a brain injury, because the nature of the injury is such that it makes you totally self-centered in your quest to rediscover and reform yourself. This self-centeredness is not a bad thing, and enables you focus on your greatest loss (self) that is to be healed. You may not feel guilt unless you were responsible for injuring others, or are aware of abandoning loved ones due to your injuries.

Remedy for Guilt

When you ask yourself *"If only I had done_____?"* you place yourself precisely in the moment of decision, and give yourself the opportunity to choose again, even though you realize it doesn't change the outcome of your loss. If you get stuck on the outcome of your choice, and perceive it as negative, guilt can become an extremely paralyzing state of mind that can keep you from making any choice at all through perceiving yourself as the source of all bad choices. It is better to keep your choices fluid and practice guilt in a limited way.

Re-living your choice in the matter of a loss is internal work and can go a long way towards helping you process it. Whether or not you made the right choice is something that you will have to leave to the future to find out, because you never know how you will evolve through your experience.

Acceptance

Acceptance of a loss does not signify that the pain has gone away. It only refers to a level of pain that is tolerable and has become mild enough to be part of your comfort level.

Acceptance and Brain Injury

With brain injury, acceptance means that you have become *relatively* comfortable with the reflections of yourself that the world is giving back to you. Before your injury you were completely comfortable with the reflections you were getting back from the world about who you were. You may not have liked the reflections that you were getting back before your injury, but you knew where they were coming from—even if you felt your intentions were misread. At least you felt that the misread intentions were yours. Now, after your injury, you are getting back reflections about yourself that are not connected to any image that you are familiar with.

Acceptance of your new self-image is not only dependent upon completion of the grieving process, but also dependent upon years of learning to live with yourself as a new person. This process includes the passing through of a number of stages including long and confusing period of *false starts*.

CHAPTER 4

False Starts

In the process of recovering from a brain injury, a false start is evidence that you are busy rebuilding yourself and just haven't found the right path yet. This vital part of your process gives you the opportunity to try out various aspects of your new self, which are yearning to become strong enough to make impressions on your self-image. This long and subtle process usually takes place in the early middle to latter stages of your healing process (3–15 years).

Looking Back

Before you have come to terms with the fact that you will never be like you were before your brain injury, you will probably try to resume your life where you left off. If you do not have the physical ability to even try to get back to your previous activities, you will constantly think about doing so—and try to realize them with your mind.

Doing What You Did Before

Trying to do what you did before will always result in disappointment because, even though you may retain some basic skills, you have changed and gotten out of step with your life. You have probably also suffered damage that has left you with less ability to do whatever it was you did before. Attempting to do what you did before your injury is a false start. It can bring you face to face with painful loss. In spite of this you must plod ahead through the grief and keep trying until you discover the right road back to yourself.

Leaping Ahead

Another, and much more treacherous type of false start is the one which springs upon you as a hopeful leap into the development of new talents. You may be sparked by visions of yourself in a new and exotic role in life, and strike out in search of ways to make this new role part of your emerging self.

Trying Something New

Don't consider it a waste of time or energy to try out new approaches to being yourself—even though they may fizzle out and leave you with an empty feeling. They are part of your process of finding yourself again. Don't forget, you did not become the person you *were* without some risk and lots of trial and error—a natural mode of achieving a goal.

You may find yourself saying *"I finally feel real," "like I fit," "excited," or "alive for the first time since my injury"* in hopes that you have broken through to being yourself again. It is important to feel good about your progress, and your excitement may be short lived. If it is, do not despair. You are just trying out new approaches to being yourself and experiencing the first rush of identification. These new roles will probably become part of you future identity—but not in the way you first conceived of them. Since they are connected to your hopes and dreams, they will become part of the image that defines you.

There is no magic path that will guide you back to feeling like your old self. Remember, the closest you can hope for is feeling comfortable with your new self.

CHAPTER 5

The Problems of a Lawsuit

This chapter is only meant to be read if your injury was the result of another's actions, and you are seeking compensation from other parties (usually insurance companies) through the legal/court systems. It is also applicable if your case is settled out of court, because part of the procedure of settling a case is usually through legal channels.

Ethical Dilemma

If you are involved in a lawsuit and are seeking recompense for personal injury, you may find yourself in a situation that is pulling you two ways at once. Your lawyer may tell you that you have to continue to look as injured as you claim to be because you may be under surveillance by insurance company investigators. It also makes common sense to keep looking injured to make a case that wins you the maximum award possible from the parties responsible for your injuries. This is not as simple as it sounds because the practical need to show your injuries, as fixed in time, is at direct odds with the progressive nature of your healing process. It also presents you with a troubling ethical problem.

The conflict you find yourself in is not of your own creation, but derives from society's use of the adversarial system to settle personal injury legal claims. Hopefully, the legal system is evolving to a point where it does not stand in the way of your innate need to heal and show progress.

Counting on a Settlement

With your life as devastated as it is due to your injuries, you are probably banking on a large settlement to help you get back on your feet. This is understandable and I don't mean to take that hope from you by encouraging you to act as healthy as you feel, no matter who is watching.

Money is extremely important, and can pay for a lot of rehabilitation. If you have suffered a loss, you deserve as much of it as you need. It is *not* in your best interest to trade your natural impulse to heal for a few extra bucks, by acting less healthy than you really are. Your job is to regain your health so that you can restore yourself and put an end to your suffering as soon as possible. Hang in there, and have faith that you will receive exactly what you need to reclaim and continue your life—even if it is not as much money as you hoped for.

Faith in a positive outcome may sound impossible to achieve if you are being squeezed for money and fighting for your life at the same time. It is difficult not to perceive those responsible for injuring you as the bad guys. *There are no bad guys here*—only rotten circumstances, irresponsible actions of self or others, or pure bad luck. You would never wish this hell of confusion and helplessness on yourself—so obviously *you* are not to blame. I believe that your life has a hidden pattern and it is best to look at your experience as the unfolding of your individual potential.

How Much is Your Injury Worth?

You might believe that winning your lawsuit will give you enough money to "put you back like you were". *No amount of money will return you to your pre-injury state of being.* Do not be fooled by a legal profession that would have you believe that the proper reward can put you back like you were.

The Scales of Justice

The law has to believe in its ability to serve justice in a quantifiable way because *it uses money to measure how much damage you have sustained at the hands of responsible parties.* Therefore it seeks to make things right by giving you back the amount it calculates you have lost. This is indeed a noble intention and can come nowhere near the mark of being able to describe your loss—especially if you have had a brain injury.

How do you put a dollar value on your perception of yourself and how you function in life? You can't!—and if you tried, you might make it more money than exists in the world. Your loss is qualitative and only you, not some court, will know when you have been restored enough to health to not want or need compensation. This time of "complete" restoration will probably not come in the three to five years most cases take to settle.

Living in Limbo

While you wait for the settlement of your lawsuit, you may feel that you are *living in limbo.* This can be an extremely unsettling part of your recovery. You will find the source of your discomfort is the attachment you are building to the outcome of your lawsuit.

Limbo Club

If you find yourself living in limbo, look for others who perceive themselves to be in the same place and start a *limbo club.* Their company and shared experience can be very comforting and help you feel more real as you water down attachments to your own projected future by empathizing with theirs. A group also gives you something to do while you wait. Local head injury support groups are a good place to start searching for others who share your experience.

Winning or Losing

When your lawsuit finally settles, you may or may not feel satisfied with the amount of money you have been awarded. If you are satisfied, you may either blow your money on impulsive attempts to buy back your old life, or use it to support more realistic and satisfactory programs of further rehabilitation (including therapy, education and tools).

If you lose your lawsuit, or don't get what you think you deserve, you may experience rage or depression as a result of your bitter disappointment. You probably won't be able to handle it alone, and I recommend that you seek counseling through contact with trusted friends, family or professionals to help you through your crisis.

Whatever the result of your court case it cannot do much to affect the long term outcome of your return to yourself. You will either find yourself as a person who got what they deserved or didn't. In either case, it is how much like yourself you feel in the long run that counts, whether you win or lose.

CHAPTER 6

Complications and Setbacks

You will experience many setbacks in your recovery process because that is the nature of healing. These setbacks will be physical, psychological, or both, and can temporarily discourage you in your hopes of becoming whole again. They will challenge you and may bring on debilitating symptoms that can appear to rob you of your progress. Don't despair! These challenges, great though they may be, have arrived at precisely the right time to help you to unfold and develop the particular strengths you need to realize the path back to yourself.

Physical Setbacks

Physical setbacks often accompany recovery from brain injury, because many brain injuries are sustained in physically invasive accidents. Therefore other parts of your body are likely to be damaged—some seriously so. If you have sustained other injuries to your body in combination with your brain injury, you are probably experiencing symptoms and treatments that are competing for your energy to heal, and contributing to a state of exhaustion and confusion.

Give Yourself a Break

Give yourself the same consideration that you would give to an injured friend or loved one, who needs the time and care to heal, and don't be taken in by the feeling that you are separated from yourself and don't really care what happens to you. Say to yourself, "*My* _____ *is injured (or broken) and needs time to heal.*"

Remedy for Lost Body Parts

It may be especially difficult to relate to physical symptoms that are a result of neurological damage because one of the most common problems with these affected areas of your body is that they don't feel like they belong to you! This disturbing state of affairs is best dealt with by consciously trying to reestablish contact with your foreign body part. If damage to the neuro-pathways that connect it to your brain is not too great, it will slowly come back to you over time. If damage is too great, the distance between you and it will remain for the rest of your life, and you will have to get used to relating to a foreign part of your body. Give it a name: "*Stupid*_____", "*Honest* _____", "_____ *with a mind of its own*"—whatever expresses best how you feel about it. *Don't forget it is part of you—even if it doesn't feel like it.*

In any case, I highly recommend that you work with a professionally trained physiotherapist to help recover use of physically disabled parts of your body. I also recommend working with a professional occupational therapist to help you connect your physical progress with the restoration of your independence. *Professional therapists need to be aware that you, as a survivor of brain injury, have a particular problem with connecting the damaged part of your body to your self-image.*

Seizures, Medication, Lack of Sleep

Unforeseen problems due to the development of seizures, reaction to medication, or sleep deprivation, can cause tremendous distress and negatively affect your emotional state because they are easily perceived as stopping your progress and putting you even further back in your healing process. There is nothing more devastating than having the feeling that you will take even longer to heal in a healing process that seems to have no end in sight.

Seizures

Seizures do not always happen after an injury to the brain, but remain a real possibility. They sometimes show up as late as one year post-injury and can usually be successfully treated with medication or alternative therapies. Your doctor or neurologist is your best resource to help you deal with seizures.

Epilepsy support groups are a good place to get information about alternative therapies that may suit your particular needs and lifestyle, but check them out with your doctor. Seizures come in various forms, ranging from mild discomfort and disorientation, to severe physical and mental disablement.

Medication

Problems relating to adjustment of medication can feel even more insurmountable than the condition they are prescribed to remedy. This is because medications often prescribed to help neurological conditions have side effects that can negatively influence your emotions. You may find yourself feeling more out of control of your emotions then you did before taking medication, and this can send you into a downward spiral of depression that will further cripple your efforts to heal.

Remember that adjusting to medication is a *process* that includes you and your doctor. Make sure that you tell your doctor if think you are experiencing negative side effects to any medication that he or she has prescribed. Hold your ground if you think you are being wrongly diagnosed by being told that "it is all in your head", and try to view medical setbacks, especially the serious ones, as temporary. They are part of your healing process. *Some day you will look back on them as if they were a bad dream.*

Lack of Sleep

You will find that you don't sleep like you used to. This can be for at least three good reasons.

First of all, brain injury is known to change your circadian rhythms. These are the physiological and behavioral patterns associated with the earth's rotation: the same ones that are disturbed when you get jet lag.

Secondly you may tend to spend your unwelcome waking hours contemplating your losses and how you got the way you are. This is part of your grieving process and a possible function of your injury related tendency to perserverate (mentally chew things over and over). It is not a bad idea to contemplate your past and might be better done during a fixed amount of time. Consciously program yourself to think about your situation for only one or two hours each day or night. Do this by saying to yourself: "I am going to *really* think about my situation for the next _____ hours *and stop when the time is up!*"

A third reason for feeling exhausted after a brain injury, is that *you are expending a great amount of energy to heal.* Consequently you are tired from all the work. Knowing why you are tired may help you go lighter on yourself and not waste your energy giving yourself grief over being tired all the time.

Loss of sleep is a great problem with brain injury and needs to be dealt with before it becomes a disabling pattern that seriously interferes with your healing process. Consultation with your doctor about medication, and referral to sleep clinics to help you sleep is highly recommended, but sleeping medication and clinics don't always work. There are experts, in the field of sleep deprivation who can help you find your sleep through the use of alternative therapies such as biofeedback and meditation. You may want to seek them out, if medication fails to help you.

If the therapies you have sought out to help you sleep fail to produce satisfactory results, you may have to learn to accept the fact that your sleeping patterns have permanently changed, and that you will never be able to regain what you perceive to be a normal and adequate amount of sleep. The best way to deal with this perception about your sleep is to *learn how to manage the sleep you do get* by taking naps, changing your schedule to accommodate your available energy, and pacing yourself. This may mean restructuring your life to reflect the limitations of your new way of being. Again I recommend consulting professionals such as counselors, physical and occupational therapists to help you make best use of your available energy.

Cognitive Setbacks

After a brain injury you will find that your brain doesn't work the way it used to. It may take longer and be more difficult for you to process your thoughts than it was before. This is because, due to your injuries, *your brain is not as neurologically flexible as it used to be.* Flexibility comes from the Latin word *"flectere"* which means to bend, and has come to mean, more specifically, the ability to bend *without breaking.* Most of us have been able to *automatically* adjust to changes in our lives, planned or not, without "breaking" under their accompanying stress on our ability to function. It is the loss, from brain injury, of the *automatic* part of this adjustment to change that compromises flexibility. This loss can make it difficult to plan, organize, and initiate tasks. It can also negatively affect your ability to make judgments, decisions, and communicate with others.

Regardless of the nature of your brain injury, the loss of a part of yourself, that has always been *automatic,* is bound to seriously affect your self-confidence and makes it especially frightening for you to project yourself in the future. Consequently, your ability to plan, organize, and initiate action is severely crippled. Be open to help with organizing the events that can bring your plans to reality because your ability to create workable sequences might have been compromised by your injury. There are many organizational aides available, from simple notebooks and bulletin boards, to electronic organizers and computers, to help you with the task of organizing your world. Occupational therapists are your best resource for obtaining these items because they are trained to provide specialized aides for specialized needs—and to teach you how to use them.

Overcoming Setbacks

Whether you have had a brain injury or not, fear, grief, and lack of self-confidence would cripple your ability to initiate action. Because you have had a brain injury, you have all three stacked against you, not to mention the results of any accompanying physical disablements. The best way to get started on anything is to *just do it*—or be on the receiving end of a good kick in the butt. "Just doing it" takes an incredible amount of courage and faith in the outcome of your action plan—if you are fortunate enough to have one. A "good kick in the butt" from a loved one, or advocate, may cause uncomfortable anxiety, but can also serve to push you past your own limitations.

You, and only you, know what you need to heal, but you may not be the best judge of *how* to get your needs met. Consult with your loved ones and advocates to help you weigh the pros and cons of your projected yearnings.

Manifesting Action Plans

Even after consultation with your supporters, you may find it extremely difficult to make decisions about how to manifest your action plans because the nature of your injury might have impaired your brain's ability to settle on one side of a question, or because you have lost the ability to pace yourself and may suffer tremendous anxiety over contemplating the unknown.

Communicating your plans to others might be difficult because of the strength of your emotion and the pressing need to see the results of your projections immediately. Remember that your healing process is a very slow one, and that the hope you have placed in the outcome of your plans may eventually help create a reality that gives you what you want, but not in the manner you have imagined.

Metaphor of Course Correction

At this, or any, stage of your recovery, it is helpful to keep in mind the metaphor of *course correction*. Course Correction is best explained through the example of "steering" a sailboat. If you are in control of the wheel or tiller of a sailboat, you have the ability to change the direction of the boat by moving the rudder. In this position of control you can direct where you want the boat to go by sighting the prow of the boat on a distant landmark or goal. Because of the countless variables of current, wind, slack in rigging or sail, and even the less than rock solid nature of your human hold on the controls, you will find yourself, moving off target to one side or the other. This can be *corrected* by adjusting the rudder to set you back in the direction of your goal. This is a process of continually aiming and correcting until you eventually get to where you are going. Course correction can be effectively used as a metaphor for any progressive action you are undertaking—especially the process of recovery from a brain injury.

CHAPTER 7

Finding Your New Self

You may feel very discouraged after experiencing false starts and battling your way through setbacks. Worse yet, you may feel that your life has no direction, and that you will never get started on the right path. It is at this point that you are most ready to challenge your limitations, and enter the part of your recovery that will have the most real effect on the re-creation of your sense of yourself as a person in the world—a vision quest. Through this quest you can discover what changes you can make to reflect the new person that you have become.

Choosing Your Path

The best way to know which path to follow is to pay attention to your strongest yearnings. These yearnings are trustworthy indicators of what it is *you* really want to do and will guide you to a proper course of action.

Yearning for Your Self

You may find yourself repeating: "*If I could only be _____ (a particular place)—then I would know what to do*", or "*If I were only given the chance to_____ (perform a particular act), then I would get better*". These statements are true indicators of your ability to perceive yourself as a whole person. Don't take them literally, but try to formulate a plan that will get you as close to your yearnings as possible. Your quest need not involve physical travel, but may be a journey of the mind directed by a knowledgeable and trusted guide.

It may not seem prudent to your caretakers for you to be carrying on about wanting to do things that they perceive are well beyond your present ability, but I believe that it is especially these requests that need to be seriously addressed. They come from your deepest faith in your potential to recover, and consequently give the most accurate clues to a path that will provide you with the most therapeutic activity.

You can be expected to have a very difficult time realizing the yearnings that you feel are driving you to action, but there will come a time, in your healing process, when they will become the next thing do. This may come about because you have directly indicated to your caregivers that you are ready and they are willing to take a shared risk and responsibility for your quest.

Starting Out on Your Vision Quest

You are now ready to go on a vision quest to find yourself. You have been on an "image" quest ever since you came to consciousness after your injury. What is the difference between an "image" quest and a "vision" quest? The difference can be found by comparing the words "image" and "vision". An "image" is a representation or *reflection* of a thing and *not* the thing itself. "Vision" is the *ability to realize it within yourself*. It is now time to exercise your *ability* to fulfill your yearning for wholeness.

Self and Self-Image

It is vitally important to understand the relationship between your "self" and your "self-image" before you start on a vision quest so that you don't waste your energy looking for the wrong thing. *Your will never find your self-image without finding your self first, because self-image is a reflection of the self.*

Searching for Your Self

Going off in search of your self takes courage and you will be more likely to achieve your goal if you don't get sidetracked by other people's fears. If family and friends think you are being reckless, then ask your professional guides to help you work out a plan.

If your quest involves travel, see if you can find someone to go with you who really loves you or is educated enough about your condition to help you through the rough spots. They have to be prepared to support you when you start falling apart, and let you suffer through the fears and disappointments that will challenge your ability to keep on going. Treat your vision quest as you would treat any new endeavor. This is especially difficult to understand if you are going to what used to be familiar territory. You will probably experience some grief as you discover that you don't even fit in your old world anymore. It is full of reflections of your old reality and not really what you went on your vision quest to find.

Being There

After you have unsuccessfully tried to fit into your old world, you may feel yourself in a state of crisis and curiously open to receive instructions that will set you off in a new and lifesaving direction. This is when it is best to be by yourself so that you can receive your first true message without distraction. *Don't forget a pen and paper or tape recorder if you have problems with your memory.*

The Right Place

Seek out, or let yourself be guided to, a place where you feel that you can be quiet and clear enough inside to hear or see what you must do to reclaim your life. This can be a special sanctuary, or nature spot where you used to go for peace and quiet, or it can be *any* new or old spot that you are drawn to in your present journey.

When you actually get to your destination, remember that you have come a long way, against great odds, to be where *you* feel you need to be to heal. Try to shut out all doubts that you are not at the right time and place in your life. You are.

Be Still

Do not be surprised at the instructions that you receive from yourself. Ask that they are for the highest good of you and those around you.

Hearing Your Self

This is your new self talking clearly, for the first time, and you are not expected to be familiar with its voice and manner. You have put your life on the line in your vision quest, and now is the time to listen.

Getting The Message

The message may be short and clear, or long and detailed, but it will always be true. This is a vital turning point in your recovery, and you have earned it by having the courage to seek it. Be sure that you have got it right before you disconnect from your point of contact. It is now your job to carry this message back to the world of your rehabilitation, and the people responsible for helping you.

Following Instructions

Coming home with inspired instructions about how to reclaim your life can make you feel like you finally know where your life is going. It can also be frightening because it may set you up to directly challenge your disabilities. This is one of those times when a very good choice can be disguised as a turn down the wrong path. Have faith in your inspired instructions, they are really all you have to guide you back to experiencing yourself as a whole person.

Sharing Your Plans

Translating your newfound plans into action may cause family and caregivers to either get excited and jump on the bandwagon to help you to get going, or project their fears for you and try to hold you back in old patterns of helplessness. Either way, you will be faced with a direct challenge to advocate for yourself, because the true product of a vision quest is most closely aligned with *your* unfolding.

You will know that you are on the right track when you discover that your newfound plans are unfolding with little or no resistance—like they are "meant to be". Having this experience does not necessarily mean that you have plugged into a supernatural state of grace, but rather that you are reclaiming responsibility for your own actions.

Beginning Again

Once you have dedicated yourself to set your inspired instructions into action, and organize the support necessary, you may feel a bit disconnected from yourself as if you are living in a dream. This is because *you are crossing the boundary between feeling and acting like your old self and feeling and acting like your new self.* You can count on the momentum of your healing process to carry you through this transition—even though the feeling of getting in step with the emergence of your new life may have a disturbing sense of unreality about it.

Learning to Feel Real

Everything may seem new to you and you will find yourself looking more to the props and costumes of your life to feel real, than to your feelings about what you are doing. This, again, is an indication of the re-stimulation of your self-image.

It is good to remember that nobody else is looking as closely at you, than you are yourself. It is your primary psychological job to be self-conscious, and you will be better off if you learn to accept it as part of what you need to do to recover.

Asking for Help

This is a good time to engage the help of specialized professionals, such as counselors and psychologists, who are trained to help you translate your vision for yourself from inspiration to reality based plans of action. These plans might include the exploration of further assessment and/or appropriate work placement, training or education.

CHAPTER 8

Starting Your New Life

Now that you feel fortified by the knowledge that you have received true instruction from a deep and fundamental source, you are ready to begin to create a new and different way of being in the world. This does not mean that you have to recreate yourself as a completely new person, and start to build a new personality from scratch. It only means that a part of you, that was not visible in your old self-image, and consequently not there for you to define yourself by, is becoming available to be incorporated into your new idea of who you are.

The process of recreating yourself as a new person involves a lot of courage to explore the new territory that you have set out for yourself in your vision. It is scary to set off to perform as a competent person when you don't quite feel like one yet. You will also need to be able to accept, what you may perceive as, limitations of abilities and talents that are a negative result of your injuries. Following your inspired instructions is not as easy as it looks from the euphoric viewpoint of just having received them. It is a slow, arduous and sometimes painful process of discovery.

Following Through on Your Plan

The best way to overcome your fear of not being able to follow through on your inspired plan of regaining your life is to go back to the point of inspiration that you experienced and re-live it in your mind. The strength of this experience should be strong enough to overcome any doubts seeded and created by an outside world that has been assessing and describing you through quantifiable eyes.

Neuropsychological Examination

A neuropsychological examination and report, administered and prepared by a qualified neuropsychologist, can be one of the most devastating reflections that you will get from your post injury world. It can come well before your vision quest or after. Whenever it comes, don't rush to read it. Wait until you think you are strong enough to hear negative things about your condition.

Being Examined

The experience of being examined, like a laboratory rat, with the expressed purpose of trying to find out what is wrong with you, may turn you off so badly that you will want nothing more than to run screaming from the testing room. The tests themselves are designed to ferret out your deficits and may be extremely frustrating. Frustration and anxiety are often normal responses to being put under scrutiny, and are probably exaggerated in survivors of brain injury because of the resulting lack of self-confidence.

Be honest with your examiner as to how you feel about being tested, for you will find that many professionals in this field are aware of how offensive the necessary procedures of their task may seem to you, and are willing to work with you to make them less so.

Interpreting Your Exam

Neuropsychological reports are sometimes prepared for the benefit of insurance companies, lawyers, and other professionals who might not really care about you and your feelings. It is important to keep this in mind when trying to decide if you, or your family really want to read these *seemingly* condemning and pessimistic views of your post injury abilities. The reading of your report is not to be taken lightly. Don't read it unless you have been prepared by a knowledgeable professional who can interpret it in the most positive, helpful, and yet realistic light. Make sure that you trust and feel good about the person you choose for this task.

Remember, it is you, and not the professionals, who are at the center of your recovery and healing process. A neuropsychological report, no matter how condemning it may seem upon first reading, can be full of helpful and supportive information that you may not be able to understand until you have attempted to realize the work laid out for you in your advanced recovery plans. At this point you may be thankful for the forewarnings of your earlier tests. They can help you know more about your condition, and give you a better ability to explain problems related to your disabilities to family, caretakers, co-workers, and bosses—and sometimes even to yourself.

Living With Disability

You may have to learn to live with visible and invisible disabilities that are a result of your injury. There is a great difference between these two states and you may be left with one or the other—or both to deal with.

Visible Disability

Visible disabilities, no matter how gross or subtle, will always stand out in your mind as a giant billboard that says to others: "See me, I'm a gimp!" This can be extremely painful—especially when your pre-injury image of yourself was that of a vital and healthy person. In your quest to reclaim yourself as a fully functioning person, anything less than appearing healthy is a mortal blow to your self-confidence and esteem.

It is unfortunate that we are trained by our culture to perceive our own, and others wholeness by how we present to view. Anything other than a healthy presentation is cause for an individual to see him or her self as less than whole, and consequently, less than fully valued as a human being. Therefore, when you have a visible disability, such as a speech impediment or mobility/motor problem, you can't help but be aware that you are being viewed as less than whole.

Counteracting Negative Self-Perception

The best way to counteract this negative perception of yourself is to keep in mind that you are actually *greater* than a whole because you are involved in the process of healing, and the very act of healing, as an inevitably positive process, can *add* to the perception of yourself as a human being *in process*.

Don't forget that everyone is in the process of healing from any number of visible or invisible, psychological/cognitive or physical assaults to their equilibrium—no matter how healthy they may present to view.

Invisible Disability

Invisible disabilities are sometimes much more confounding than visible ones because the world expects you to have the ability to function fully if you look like you can. This gross misjudgment of ability is a form of cultural blindness that is paradoxically caused by the overemphasis we put on appearance.

Ability cannot be generalized to all challenges and tasks. Your ability to competently meet a challenge and carry out a task is specific to that task and its attendant variables. Because you have suffered a brain injury you are not automatically disabled in all things. You will retain many abilities, and suffer the loss of others.

Memory Problems

Invisible problems with memory are injury specific and vary greatly from injury to injury making it impossible and insulting to generalize and predict how they can affect specific situations. When working to restore your memory, with or without professional help, it is best to concentrate on rebuilding your world with memories or flashes of memory that are *important to you* regardless of how bizarre they may seem to others. *It is your mind and you own it* no matter how others may try to channel it into what makes sense to them. The most effective strategies for recovery of your memory are consequently best worked out and refined by you as you discover and learn through experience the specific nature of your deficits. You may want to engage the help of specialized counselors or psychologists to gain access to aids and programs that most effectively address your needs.

Cognitive Problems

Invisible cognitive difficulties can negatively affect sequencing, multi-tasking, organization, and speed of processing. The fact that you perceive the world in a concretely unique and different way from others, makes it all the more important that you *develop your own specific strategies* to deal with loss of memory and ability to function in time and space.

You may be called upon to perform tasks that have become extremely difficult or virtually impossible for you. It is inevitable that you will feel great frustration in being expected to do things that you literally can't do—or can't do up to the standards expected. The best way to deal with this situation and avoid the misguided and painful criticism and self-depreciation that can easily follow is to learn about your invisible disabilities and how they affect your ability to function.

Since you are the one experiencing the disability, no one knows better what it feels like than you, so no professional expert, caregiver, or family member, regardless of his or her training or closeness to you, can accurately speak for you. He or she can however help you communicate the uniqueness of your situation. *Therefore your helper must be educated by you to understand your invisible limitations.*

Communicating Your Frustration

Your level of frustration and grief over being misunderstood and not being able to perform like you think you should, may make it difficult for you to take on this task of education by yourself. Use this book and anyone you respect as a trusted advocate and communicator to help you with this task. Above all *be honest with your feelings* and have patience with those trying to understand and help you. Remember, they have no idea what you are going through!

CHAPTER 9

Post Traumatic Stress And Related Symptoms

Post Traumatic Stress has found its way, as a qualified disorder, into the pages of the Diagnostic and Statistical Manual of the American Psychiatric Association. It has more to do with the way that trauma is related to memory than most other specified disorders. Consequently it is often associated with survivors of brain injury.

Because of its obvious cause and effect nature, Post Traumatic Stress is not difficult to figure out. It requires the particular understanding that we are only able to commit to memory that which we have a story for. If, for some reason, we have been so traumatized by an event that we can't, or won't think of it as a story, trauma, finding no refuge in memory, hides itself in the very fabric of our experience. There, it lurks waiting to be triggered so that it can overtake our reality and literally force us to re-live the original horror we experienced. The experience of re-living a trauma, without a story to protect us from its devastating emotional effects, is terrifying and lies at the very core of a Post Traumatic Stress episode

The scary part is that you never know what will trigger an episode or when you will have the intrusive dreams, flashbacks, or disturbing patterns of avoidance, and feelings of dread coupled with unaccountable physical distress, that are symptoms associated with Post Traumatic Stress. It is also sometimes difficult to separate symptoms of your positive healing process from those of Post Traumatic Stress. Part of your job, in healing is to learn to distinguish which symptoms are a function of your positive healing process, and which are the debilitating symptoms of Post Traumatic Stress.

Dreams

Seemingly intrusive dreams may be associated with a damaged memory trying to restore and make sense of a shattered world as it re-connects and re-patterns pre and post injury experience. They may also be symptoms of Post Traumatic Stress.

Dreaming About Your Old Life

Some of your dreams may be more recurrent than intrusive and demand your attention because of their insistent repetitiveness. Repetition of a dream, especially one about your life *as it was before,* is likely to be an indication of your self-image working to create a new image that is more easily blended with your pre-injury past. This is a great task and it is no wonder that you are involved in it twenty–four hours a day. Dreams provide a comprehensive environment for the creation of your new self with easily adjustable components of your old and new perception of reality.

You may find yourself dreaming about your old life over and over for many years after your injury. As time goes on, you will notice, in your dreams, that elements of your old world begin to transform into landmarks associated with your new one. When this happens reoccurring dreams will cease to feel less intrusive and become more affirmative of a new sense of well being in the world. This transformation of your dreams from uncomfortable to affirming is an indication of the deeper reestablishment of your self-image and can be looked at as a good sign in your healing process.

Intrusive Dreams About Trauma

If you find that your reoccurring dreams are more connected to events immediately or closely surrounding your trauma than cherished aspects of your old life, you may be experiencing a symptom of Post Traumatic Stress. These dreams are also noticeably uncomfortable and continue to negatively affect your emotional state after awakening. They are a manifestation of your need to come to terms with the experience of your trauma and are best dealt with through therapy designed to uncover and recover memory of buried trauma.

Flashbacks

Flashbacks to old life

Flashbacks to events that are connected with your old life are most likely part of the same process of rebuilding your self-image as the first type of recurrent dreams mentioned above. As such they may be more comforting and hopeful than disturbing and intrusive. This is because the sense of reality usually conveyed in a flashback is convincingly real. It may also be a symptom of Post Traumatic Stress.

When you feel real about an aspect of your old life, you have a fleeting sense of yourself as a real person in the world. This can produce a sense of magically returning to how you used to be before your brain injury.

Do not be fooled by this type of flashback. You will never be like you were before—different, maybe even better than before,—but never the same. The frequency of this type of flashback will diminish as your self-image heals and reestablishes itself. Being aware of the reduction of flashbacks is useful in helping you keep faith in your positive progress.

Disturbing Flashbacks

Flashbacks of bits and pieces of experience that are difficult to recognize and have a distinctly invasive or violent nature are probably a symptom of Post Traumatic Stress. Like invasive dreams associated with Post Traumatic Stress, these flashbacks are an indication of your need to come to terms with the experience of your trauma, and are best dealt with through therapy designed to uncover and recover memory of buried trauma.

Deja Vue

You can have a third type of flashback that is more like a *deja vue* experience than anything else. This flashback is not like the *deja vue* you may have felt at other times in your life. It can be distinctly disorienting and feel like it is taking over your whole reality. Flashbacks of this nature are sometimes indicative of abnormal neurological activity in your brain, including auras that precede seizures, and other symptoms from your injury that indicate neurological damage to your brain. These flashbacks should be reported to your physician/neurologist and are usually treatable if they get in your way.

Avoidance

Patterns of avoidance of particular places, things or situations may be due to your inability to face your losses or a distinct symptom of Post Traumatic Stress. It seems obvious that you might want to avoid anything that rubs your nose in aspects of your life that you believe are lost forever. Nobody wants that kind of pain! You also don't want to be around anything that triggers the extremely uncomfortable symptoms of Post Traumatic Stress.

Avoidance and Loss

Avoiding particular places, things, and situations to keep from facing your losses can be seen as a secondary function of denial and as such is part of your healing process from loss. Don't let anyone force or push you too fast into situations that evoke intense grief.

Take your time and respect the needs of your natural grieving process as a powerful therapeutic tool that is created and administered by you, and you alone. This is important! Remember, again, that *you are the ultimate judge of how quickly, and in what manner you need to heal!*

Avoidance of things and situations that greatly repel you makes sense if you don't want those feelings. It can also be a sure sign that you are being triggered by whatever you are avoiding and experiencing symptoms of Post Traumatic Stress. If these patterns of avoidance are standing in the way of your pursuing or maintaining a life situation that you know is good for you, you may wish to seek therapeutic help to come to terms with your buried trauma.

Feelings of Dread and Physical Symptoms

Neurological Symptoms?

Feelings of dread coupled with nausea, dizziness, and disorientation that spring upon you without warning can easily be confused with pre-seizure auras and other neurological symptoms.

These physical symptoms should be immediately reported to your physician/neurologist for they may be indications of life-threatening developments, such as tumors, seizures, or other neurological damage related to your injuries. These symptoms can be medically treated, and the threat to life removed, if caught in time.

The physical symptoms mentioned above can be, and often are, symptoms of Post Traumatic Stress. Something, unknown to you, in your immediate environment has triggered you to physically re-live your trauma without the comfort of a story line. This experience can be extremely debilitating and completely interrupt your life on a temporary basis.

The good news is that you, alone, can learn to deal with this most devastating symptom. The idea is to recognize the onset of these symptoms and ground yourself before they take over your consciousness.

Grounding Yourself

There are many grounding exercises available in the teachings of any number of spiritual/physical healing paths. You may have learned one in your old life, or you may have been taught one in one of your present therapies. No matter where you have learned it, it is imperative that you practice a grounding exercise that works for you *as soon as you experience any of the symptoms mentioned above.*

If you do not have a meditation of your own, here is one that I find useful to ground me when I need it.

1) *center your energy in your lower abdomen (tanden).*
2) *direct the focused energy down the front of your body—deep into the core of the earth.*
3) *draw the energy from the core of the earth up through your spine and out the top of your head—way out into the center of the universe.*
4) *return the energy from the center of the universe back down into your lower abdomen and feel it rest there to be sent again into the core of the earth where it will come up through your spine and create a circle that informs you that you are of the earth and heavens at one and the same time.*

This meditation can help you create and maintain a dynamic grounding that keeps you connected, above and below so that you are not thrown off balance by the symptoms of a Post Traumatic Stress induced episode. It, as well as other meditations or exercises you have learned, may also be helpful to keep you grounded in any situation where you want to be able to function with clear and centered energy.

CHAPTER 10

Living With Your New Self

As you can see, recovery from a serious trauma, especially one that includes a brain injury, can be an arduous and uncomfortable process. Don't let this knowledge dishearten you. You have at least three things in your favor: time, the positive nature of your healing process, and the deep-seated faith in the knowledge that you can and eventually will regain your sense of wholeness. Overcoming adversity implies that there is something to overcome, and there is no foe more treacherous than lingering remnants of your trauma and injuries.

Time Heals

You will find over time that the more you strive to become conscious of what has happened to you, the less you will be negatively affected by triggers and symptoms that used to cause you distress. Known triggers and symptoms will be less debilitating and hidden ones will become less transparent and easier to live with.

Keep Practicing

Keep practicing your grounding exercises long after you think you have vanquished any symptoms of Post Traumatic Stress you may have. These meditations can serve you well while you are reestablishing yourself as a new person—especially before and during challenges to perform concrete actions that are still difficult for you.

Remember that even though you may feel that a new self has been successfully formed, you are still going to constantly compare yourself to your pre-injury state. This is because your new image is infused with the momentum of your healing process and has not been around long enough for you to experience it as an unquestionable part of yourself. Your old self-image, however, existed *without doubt* in your pre-injury concept of yourself and will always remain as a point of comparison for you—and as a seemingly lost state of being that you will be involved in grieving for the rest of your life.

This grieving will take less and less of your energy as you become acquainted with aspects of your new self that begin to produce success-ful and gratifying relationships with the world. You may even wonder "who" it is that is achieving all the success, and experience periods of discomfort around things that you think should make you feel better.

Feeling Like a Fraud

Feeling like a fraud is an understandable outcome of reconstructing yourself and a particularity uncomfortable state of being. You were not born like this, and can no longer refer to an image of yourself that *automatically* conforms to your natural developmental patterns and experience.

Remedy for Feeling Like a Fraud

The best way to counter feeling like a fraud is to remember that the only person who feels that way about you is *yourself*. Most people take you at face value and never question whether or not *you are you*. They may only notice that you are having some discomfort and are displaying a consequent tentativeness. This is not usually enough to have you treated as an undesirable outsider—only perceived as a shy or somewhat self-conscious person.

You may, however, continue to experience distinct feelings of aloneness—especially in groups whose members tend to emphasize their similarity to each other. This is because such groups rely on the *automatic* feelings of comfort that they derive from mutual backgrounds and interests. Because you may have chosen pre-injury friendships and affiliations to match your comfort level in groups like the ones mentioned above, you will now find yourself feeling estranged from old friends and their activities.

Feeling Alone

Your brain injury, and resulting damage to self-image, may have left you without the functional background to enjoy participation in groups concentrating on activities that you were fluent in before your injury. You may choose to look upon this situation as a point to be grieved—or an opportunity to seek out and discover through the processes of elimination and trial and error new groups and associations with individuals that allow you to derive satisfaction from your life.

Be Kind to Yourself

Be careful that you don't compare yourself unfavorably with new friends, or groups who have not had the experience of having to recreate their lives. They will inevitably be able to express more confidence in their behavior than you do because it is *automatic* for them to see themselves in relation to the world.

You, on the other hand, have the unique ability to create your life as you go along and experience each moment as a new brush stroke on the canvass of your self-image.

Reclaiming Your Life

The most important point to remember, as you recreate your life, is that *you* are the artist who is painting the picture of yourself *for yourself* in your mind, even though you think you are creating it to be seen through the eyes of others. In a sense your brain injury has given you the rare opportunity to consciously recreate yourself *as you really are* and not just as how you think you want others to see you.

Conclusion

I have suffered one of the most harrowing experiences known to the human mind, (the conscious loss of self) and consider myself fortunate to be able to end this book on an optimistic note. At this point in my recovery, I can say to you with confidence, that it is more than possible to recover a full sense of personal wholeness following serious injury to the brain. After twenty years the questions of "Who am I?" and "Where am I in the world?" have finally stopped dominating my thought and robbing me of my effectiveness.

—and I have received many gifts including the unexpected return of, what I thought were, "lost" abilities.

978-0-595-20942-2
0-595-20942-4